Information
JUNKIES

presents...

STEP 3
BOARD-READY
USMLE JUNKIES

The Must-Have USMLE Step 3 Review Companion

by USMLE JUNKIES & Dr. B. Show, M.D., M.B.A

LA LA SINCERELY

Atlanta

1

First printing

This publication contains educational information in the field of medicine. Medicine is always changing especially when new research and clinical developments become available for education. The author and publisher have checked with sources to make sure information and educational material contained in this book are up-to-date to meet the standards accepted at the time of publication. Due to the possibility of human errors and updates in medicine and research and sciences, neither the author, publisher, nor contributors herein, warrants or guarantees the information contained in this book is in every aspect accurate or complete. They disclaim all warranties including without limitation any implied warranty of fitness for a particular purpose and responsibility for any errors or omissions, or for the results found in this book. For example, any medication or drug therapy mentioned herein is not to be used as guide when administering a patient, but readers are encouraged to check product information sheet and confirm with other sources.

The author and publisher specifically disclaim all responsibility for any liability, loss, or right, personal, medical, or otherwise, which is incurred as a consequence, directly or indirectly, of the use and application of any contents of this book.

LA LA SINCERELY has allowed this work to remain exactly as the author intended, verbatim, without editorial input. USMLE JUNKIES is a subsidiary of LA LA SINCERELY

When ordering this title, use ISBN: 978-0-9855124-0-8
PUBLISHED BY LA LA SINCERELY
www.usmlejunkies.com
Printed in the United States of America

LA LA SINCERELY°

Atlanta

Dedication

To the future doctors who want success and are passionate about helping others because this is their calling.

To families and friends for their understanding and support during the compilation of this book.

Acknowledgments

Thanks to the residents for their feedback and recommendations throughout the development of *Step 3 Board-Ready USMLE Junkies*.

Thanks to the editor for an outstanding work and making our job easier.

Contents

8

Introduction

This book was written to find a systematic approach to reviewing for Step 3. While there are many choices of review books out there, this review book would give you a quick glance at the subject matter while relating it to other important areas in medicine. It is more like a stepwise approach to any subject matter. There isn't any other Step 3 review book that uses a stepwise, quick, and high-yield approach in this manner.

It is obvious that before you take the Step 3 examination, you would have either taken Step 1 and 2, or you have knowledge of the examination materials already. Step 1 or Step 2 is not any easier than Step 3. However, Step 3 is probably the most important as a practicing physician because it deals with questions that are relevant to patient management both in-patient and out-patient settings.

While it is recommended you take Step 3 during or after your residency, you may still take it before residency if you're well prepared for it. *Step 3 Board-Ready USMLE Junkies* will help you achieve this success. Depending on your familiarity with the Step 3 materials, it is important to also use a comprehensive textbook along with this book, *Step 3 Board-Ready USMLE Junkies* as a supplement.

The topics found on Step 3 cover all subspecialties. The questions are multiple-choices, usually long, and mostly clinically-oriented. The Step 3 is a 2-day examination. The first day is all multiple-choice questions, and the second day is both multiple-choice questions and clinical-case scenarios, a Computer-based Case Simulations (CCS), where you examine and manage a patient in both emergency and office settings. It is important that you practice the clinical-case scenarios before attempting the Step 3 because they are crucial to the passing of this exam. The practice relies on the familiarity with the use of the CCS software.

Computer-based Case Simulations (CCS)

Practicing your case simulations is very important in order to pass the Step 3. Make sure you are familiar with the software that comes with your registration package or can be found on USMLE website. The exam is given on Day 2 of the Step examination.

Here are some tips to help with making the computer-based case simulations easier.

WHEN TO ADMIT TO ICU

Mnemonics: **DR D.E.M.S** = DKA → **R**espiratory failure → **D**elirium → **E**lectrolytes imbalance → **M**I (post) → **S**hock.

INITIAL WORKUP TO CONSIDER IN ER

Mnemonics: **V.O.I.C.E.S** = **V**itals (including cardiac & BP monitoring) → **O**xygen (& pulse **O**ximetry and/or ABG) → **I**VF (**hold off initially in CHF;** & IV access) → **C**hest x-ray → **E**CG (and Echo) → **S**ymptoms (treat presenting symptoms).

TIPS DURING EXAMINATION

When you just don't know the answer:

1. Choose the **most common cause**.
2. Remember answers that seem to be right most of the time such as: **corticosteroids/steroids (prednisone), indomethacin,** or **ACEIs**. These answers are usually there because they may be the answers. So if you don't know, they are 'safer' options.
3. Look out for 'obvious' or the 'simpliest' answer such as: **'observe', self-limiting, follow-up with serial x-rays, NPO/IVFs/Antibiotics** combination, **dietary**

history, or **medication list**.   These answers are there and can be easily overlooked; they are what we call the 'DUH moment!'

4. Be confident. Sometimes, you may need to work from your answer choices back up to the questions (instead of the questions to the answer choices). You should look at the answer choices to see in what scenario they would have been the answers. So you are using the 'unlikely' answer choices that you are sure are NOT possible to arrive at the most likely or the 'got-to-be' answer choice.

Chapter 1
Cardiology
Chest Pain and Myocardial Infarct

1. While all emergencies are considered emergency in the ER, chest pain is probably the one that requires immediate evaluation. It is a serious symptom that should be further evaluated. It calls for determining whether or not the chest pain relates to the heart.
2. It is important to remember that atherosclerotic occlusion of the coronary arteries => **primary cause of ischemic heart disease.**
3. **When you have a patient with epigastric pain, consider acute coronary syndrome = unstable angina in your diagnosis because it is the most common cause of epigastric pain.**
4. Stable angina => a patient has chest pain or shortness of breath during exertion which is relieved with rest or nitroglycerin.
5. Unstable angina => a patient has chest pain or shortness of breath during rest which is not relieved with rest or nitroglycerin.
6. Myocardial Infarction => chest pains that persist for **15-30 minutes** and may or may not **radiate to the shoulder, arm, or jaw**. Look for an ECG which shows **flipped** or **flattened T waves** and **ST-segment elevation**.
7. Don't make the mistake--some myocardial infarctions are **asymptomatic** and **silent**; therefore, they may present as atypical in some young and even elderly patients!

Lab Tests/Diagnosis:
1. Chest pain => **always** CHECK cardiac enzymes + ECG + Chest x-ray.
2. Cardiac enzymes => creatine kinase (CK-MB) **(every 8 hours X 3 times)**, troponin, lactate dehydrogenase (LDH) **(rises after 24 hours-late presentation)**.
3. Chest x-ray => may show cardiomegaly or pulmonary congestion.
4. Echocardiography => if you suspect valvular disease or congestive heart failure.
5. **THINK: C. E. C. E =>** Cardiac enzymes + ECG + Chest x-ray + Echocardiography.

Treatment:
1. **O**xygen, **N**itroglycerin, **A**spirin, **P**lavix (clopidogrel), **H**eparin, **A**CEI, **B**eta blocker, **S**tatin (and morphine for pain if pulmonary edema is present) => **THINK: ON APH ABS.**
2. **Cardiac catheterization** is used to locate occlusions and determine the severity.

Occlusion may be treated with **angioplasty** and **stent placement**.

3. Cardiac rehabilitation in the form of supervised exercise is recommended 4-6 weeks post-MI.
4. Order a cardiac stress test after 24-48 hours in a patient with chest pains (non-acute) in the following conditions: no risk factors, when the result is equivocal or the presence of coronary artery disease is uncertain with normal cardiac enzymes, and normal ECG.
5. A patient complaining of **fear of sudden death** during sexual activity **post-MI** may be due to **anxiety**. Remember also that anxiety is a more common cause of erectile dysfunction in post-MI patients than beta-blockers.
6. When a less common cause of erectile dysfunction in post-MI patients is due to beta blocker medications → just hold the drug and reevaluate!

Post Myocardial Infarction Complications:

1. Ventricular fibrillation, ventricular tachycardia, sinus bradycardia, heart block, cardiogenic shock, papillary muscle rupture, ventricular septal defect, Dressler's syndrome, and fibrinous pericarditis.
2. If **acute pulmonary edema** exists **2-5 days after an MI** => it may be due to papillary muscle rupture and mitral regurgitation. Obtain a transthoracic echocardiography or a transesophageal.

Stress Test

1. Stress test => may be used to **assess pretest probability** in patients with history of chest pains and risk factors for coronary artery disease.
2. It is also used to assess the functional capacity in patients with known coronary artery diseases.
3. Remember that in a patient with chest pain and coronary artery disease risk factors, always **obtain cardiac enzymes** to rule out MI **before** performing a **stress test**.
4. Please do **not** obtain a stress test in patients with: acute aortic dissection, aortic stenosis, third degree heart block, acute coronary syndrome, and decompensated heart failure!

Types of Stress Test:

1. **Exercise Stress Test:**
- Patient walks on treadmill, and the response to stress is evaluated on ECG.
- Indicated for patients who **can** walk or exercise **without difficulty**.
- Clinical symptoms to observe are chest pains or shortness of breaths.
- ECG changes may include ST depressions or other arrhythmias.
- Specificity is low for patients with resting ECG changes.
- Adding nuclear component to perfusion study increases sensitivity.

2. **Adenosine Stress Test/Persantine (Dipyrimadole) Test:**
- Vasodilation test helps to dilate arteries with lesions.
- Indicated for patients who **cannot** walk or exercise **with difficulty** due to → peripheral arterial disease, osteoarthritis, or obesity.
- Also indicated for patients → already on beta blocker → with left bundle branch block (LBBB) → or premature ventricular contractions (PVCs).

3. **Dobutamine Stress Test (Echocardiography):**
- Used to determine the abnormal wall and viability. Ischemic wall is hypokinetic.
- Indicated for patients with **moderate to severe COPD or asthma, third-degree heart block,** or where persantine is contraindicated.

Valvular Heart Disease
Aortic Stenosis

- Chest pain **+** syncope during **exertion + exercise intolerance +** shortness of breath with heart failure symptoms.
- Crescendo-decrescendo systolic murmur.
- **'Slow' carotid upstroke** => elderly with AS **vs 'brisk' carotid upstroke** => hypertrophic obstructive cardiomyopathy (HOCM).

Diagnosis: ECG, Chest x-ray, TTE (**best initial**), TEE (more accurate than TTE), and left heart catheterization (most accurate; measures pressure gradient; normal < 30 mmHg).	Treatment of symptomatic AS => aortic valve replacement. Use valvuloplasty in adult patients with symptomatic AS but present with comorbid conditions.

- **Avoid** nitrates (overdiuresis) and ACEIs (vasodilator) in symptomatic patients. Follow up every 6 months to 1 year for physical assessment and evaluation with serial echocardiograms for severe and symptomatic AS.

Aortic Regurgitation

- Watch for patients who are asymptomatic or become symptomatic with heart failure.
- **Wide pulse pressure,** diastolic decrescendo murmur heard best at left sternal

border.
- Look in the history for => aortic dissection, Marfan's syndrome, syphilis, aortic root disease, ankylosing spondylitis, and reactive arthritis.

THINK: W.A.R → Wide pulse pressure => Aortic Regurgitation.

Diagnosis => ECG, Chest x-ray, TTE (**best initial**), TEE (more accurate than TTE), and left heart catheterization (most accurate; measures pressure gradient; normal < 30 mmHg).	**Treatment of AR** => **ACEIs, ARBs, nifedipine**, hydralazine, or aortic valve replacement if symptomatic or in decreased EF < 55%.

Mitral Stenosis

• Watch for patients who present with hemoptysis and heart failure. Other symptoms are dysphagia, hoarseness, and AFib. • May be caused by **rheumatic fever**. Seen in immigrant and pregnant patients (due to increased plasma volume). • Diastolic rumble after an **opening snap**.	
Diagnosis => ECG, Chest x-ray, TTE (**best initial**), TEE (more accurate than TTE), and left heart catheterization (most accurate; measures pressure gradient; normal < 30 mmHg).	**Treatment of MS** => Diuretic (**best initial**); valve replacement and **balloon valvuloplasty (most effective)**. **Same treatment in pregnancy.** **THINK => Ms. HCTZ** (Ms. Hydrochlorothiazide for treatment)

Mitral Regurgitation

• Mitral regurgitation may be asymptomatic initially, and it can later present with symptoms of heart failure (dyspnea on exertion). • **Holosystolic** murmur at apex and radiating to axilla.	
Diagnosis => ECG, Chest x-ray, TTE (**best initial**), TEE (most accurate).	**Treatment of MR** => ACEIs, ARBs, or nifedine (best initial); valve replacement or repair (best diagnostic and if EF < 60%).

	THINK => Mr. Nifedipine (for treatment)
• Risk: atrial fibrillation.	

Mitral Valve Prolapse

- Mitral valve prolapse is usually asymptomatic. It may present with **palpitations**.
- MVP is associated with **panic attacks** or panic disorder.
- Endocarditis prophylaxis is **not** required for MVP.

THINK: P in Prolapse => Panic attacks → **P**alpitations.

Infective Endocarditis

1. Symptoms => **acute (infectious)**: fever, rigors, heart failure, and **neurologic problems with systemic emboli**; **subacute**: weeks to months of fever, malaise, weight loss; **noninfectious**: asymptomatic and heart failure.
2. Physical exam findings => new murmur, tenderness over the spine and focal neurologic deficits (present with septic emboli); **infectious**: painful nodules (Osler's nodes) on fingers and toes, Janeway lesions on skin, and retinal exudates (Roth's spots).
3. High risk patients => they usually have history of prosthetic heart valves, previous infective endocarditis, cyanotic congenital heart disease, surgically repaired pulmonary shunts, or are injection drug abusers.
4. **High risk procedures needing prophylaxis** in **high risk** patients => **dental procedures** such as tooth extraction, scaling and cleaning, gingival manipulation, and **respiratory procedure** such as rigid (not flexible) bronchoscopy.
5. Organisms that cause endocarditis are => subacute (most common): streptococcus viridians, enterococci, staph epidermidis, and candida. Acute: Staph Aureus in IVDA.

Lab Tests/Diagnosis:
1. **Noninfectious:** Echocardiography => incidental finding.
2. **Infectious:** Obtain three sets of blood cultures + transthoracic echocardiogram (TTE). If the latter is negative, perform transesophageal echocardiography (TEE) because it is more sensitive and it shows vegetations.
3. **ECG** (if it shows **heart block** => indicates **abscess**).

Treatment:
1. Antibiotics => nafcillin + gentamicin or vancomycin + gentamicin in IVDA. Gentamicin provides synergism.
2. **Prophylaxis** is recommended only in **high-risk patients**.
3. Prophylaxis is **not** recommended in gastrointestinal or gastrourinary procedures.
4. **Prophylaxis treatment** is a single dose of oral azithromycin or clindamycin one hour prior to the procedure or 30 minutes prior intravenously.
5. Injection drug abusers should discontinue injection drug use for preventive measures of further occurrence of infectious endocarditis.

Complications:
*   Septic emboli, acute aortic regurgitation, and aortic valve abscess.

Congestive Heart Failure

1. Most common cause => atherosclerosis.
2. Heart failure => categorized into => systolic, diastolic, valvular, and arrhythmia-causing heart failures.
3. Systolic: Heart is unable to pump well => this may be due to **ischemia and long-standing hypertension** with S3 gallop, orthopnea, and lower extremity swelling.
4. Diastolic: Heart is stiff and unable to relax and fill with blood => this may be due to hypertension with **left ventricular hypertrophy**.

Lab Tests/Diagnosis:
1. Obtain ECG and cardiac enzymes to rule out myocardial infarct.
2. Obtain echocardiography to determine ejection fraction and valvular defects.
3. Obtain chest x-ray to evaluate fluid overload.
4. Obtain TSH.

Treatment:
1. ACE inhibitor; if there's cough as a side effect, => use ARB. If angioedema and cough exist => use hydralazine + isosorbide.
2. Beta blocker (metoprolol, atenolol, or carvedilol). Use with caution in acute cases.
3. Loop diuretics (furosemide) in exacerbation.
4. Spironolactone for stage III/IV.
5. Hydralazine + Nitrates reduce mortality in African Americans.
6. Digoxin reduces morbidity (the need for hospitalizations) not mortality.
7. ACEIs + beta blockers + spironolactone => decrease mortality → they are used in long-term treatment of CHF.
8. Aspirin and statin.
9. Most common cause of death in CHF => arrhythmia → place implantable cardioverter or automatic implantable cardiac defibrillators (AICDs).

10. Indications for AICDs => **dilated cardiomyopathy, cardiogenic shock, and persistent CHF with EF < 35%**.
11. Cardiac Resynchronization Therapy (CRT) or cardiac transplantation. CRT is used in severe CHF when QRS complex > 130 msec. AICD and CRT combination reduces mortality.
12. Remember to determine the secondary cause of CHF such as MI, hypertension, atrial fibrillation, or missed dialysis, and treat the underlying cause.

Arrhythmias
Atrial Fibrillation

1. Causes vary from structural, hyperthyroidism, metabolic, CHF to alcohol.
2. Check TSH when you suspect hyperthyroidism.
3. For **stable** patients who are **symptomatic** → **control the ventricular rate** with medications → such as metoprolol, diltiazem, or verapamil. Digoxin and amiodarone may also be used to control rate.
4. For **unstable** patients who are **symptomatic** → use emergency cardioversion.
5. A patient is considered **unstable**, and **need cardioversion**, when presented with symptomatic hypotension, congestive heart failure resistant to treatment, hypoxia, and angina.
6. For acute **asymptomatic** patients → no specific treatment is needed.
7. Anticoagulate in chronic cases with **heparin and warfarin.**
8. Atrial fibrillation existing for 48 hours or more should be evaluated with TEE before cardioversion to rule out thrombus and prevent risk of stroke.
9. If thrombus is present and AFib is 48 hours or more, anticoagulate first for 3 weeks with warfarin → cardiovert → then continue warfarin for another 4 weeks.
10. For patients with Atrial fibrillation + CHF → control the rate first with metoprolol + digoxin → then with furosemide → if pulmonary edema exists, treat with morphine → if patient is decompensating, cardiovert.

Lone Atrial Fibrillation

1. Must be able to differentiate this from atrial fibrillation. This is paroxysmal atrial fibrillation.
2. This is atrial fibrillation alone without the risk factors for stroke.
3. Treatment is determined by grading using CHADS2 score. The score is used to determine the risk for stroke. CHADS2 => CHF, Hypertension, Age > 75, Diabetes, and Stroke or Transient Ischemic Attack (TIA). Each risk factor gets a score of 1 except for Stroke or TIA which gets a score of 2.
4. A patient with total **CHADS2 score of 1 or more** → **treated with warfarin**. A

score of 0 or less → treated with **aspirin only**.
5. Note: a patient with CHADS2 score of 1 or more and presents with high risk of hemorrhaging → treat this patient with aspirin only instead of warfarin.
6. In patients with AFib, risk of stroke increases if any of these risk factors also exist: increasing age, rheumatic fever, hypertension, previous MI, previous stroke, CHF, enlarged left atrium, or left ventricular dysfunction.

Ventricular Tachycardia

1. Look out for V-Tachycardia that may present as **wide complex tachycardia**.
2. Diagnosis: ECG; if negative, monitor with telemetry. Most accurate diagnostic test is with electrophysiological testing.
3. If patient has **no pulse** → treat with shock → epinephrine → shock → vasopressin → then shock again. (Notice here that you shock first before treatment).
4. Alternative treatment is with amiodarone, lidocaine, procainamide, or magnesium.

THINK: Treatment => L.A.M.P => Lidocaine → Amiodarone → Magnesium → Procainamide.
- **Tx of ventricular tachycardia => lidocaine**; however, when it is **associated with acute pulmonary edema** → treat with **synchronized cardioversion**.
- For acute pulmonary edema with AFib, flutter, or supraventricular tachycardia => Tx: synchronized cardioversion.

Ventricular Fibrillation

1. Symptom: Serious condition which can be seen as **sudden death**.
2. Diagnosis: ECG.
3. Can be treated as ventricular tachycardia using lidocaine, amiodarone, magnesium, and procainamide.
4. Emergency defibrillation (**un**synchronized cardioversion) => **most effective management**.

Pulseless Electrical Activity (PEA)

- May be due to drugs (such as in overdose), hypoxia, pulmonary embolism, tension pneumothorax, hypovolemia, and hypokalemia.

- Findings: patient presents with ECG indicating 'no pulse'.
- Diagnosis: ECG.
- Treatment: treat the underlying factor. Manage with epinephrine and atropine.

Wolff-Parkinson-White Syndrome (WPW)

1. Slurred upstroke – delta wave.
2. Usually due to worsening of SVT status-post the use of digoxin or calcium-channel blockers.
3. Diagnosis: ECG (observe delta wave), electrophysiological testing.
4. Treatment is with procainamide or quinidine. Long-term treatment is catheter ablation.

THINK: P in WPW => Procainamide.

Supraventricular Tachycardia (SVT)

1. Paroxysmal; stable tachycardia with palpitations +/- syncope.
2. Diagnosis: ECG; if negative, order holter monitor or telemetry.
3. Treatment is with vagal or carotid stimulation and valsalva for stable patients.
4. Adenosine or diltiazem (calcium channel blocker) can also be used. If unstable, cardiovert. For long-term management, use catheter ablation.

Sinus Tachycardia

- Usually no treatment.
- First identify the underlying cause. If no other symptoms, treat with beta blocker such as propanolol.

Premature Ventricular

Contractions (PVCs)

1. Usually no treatment.
2. If symptoms persist, treat with lidocaine.

Torsades de Pointes

1. It's a specific type of polymorphic ventricular tachycardia with undulating amplitude. Also known as **prolonged QT syndrome**.
2. Causes include hypokalemia, hypomagnesium, quinidine, macrolide (clarithromycin), psychotic drugs such as tricyclic antidepressants or phenothiazine, and alcohol.
3. Diagnosis: ECG → prolonged QT interval.
4. Management => admit to ICU → obtain ECG → if ECG changes exist, treat with **sodium bicarbonate** → if other arrhythmias exist, treat with **lidocaine** → may need to **check magnesium** level → treat with magnesium if low.

Sinus Bradycardia

1. Heart rate (HR) < 60 beats per minute (bpm).
2. If asymptomatic and HR > 40 bpm, no treatment is needed.
3. If symptomatic and HR < 60 bpm, treat with atropine first, then temporary, or permanent pacemaker if needed.
4. If < 40 bpm and patient is either asymptomatic or symptomatic, treat with atropine + temporary or permanent pacemaker. **ANY HEART RATE BELOW 40 SHOULD BE ADDRESSED with a pacemaker.**
5. Medications such as calcium channel and beta blockers must be avoided to prevent further slowing of HR.

Heart Blocks

- History (such as tick bites, digoxin toxicity, beta blocker, calcium channel blocker, lupus, etc.) and physical examination (such as atrophy) may hint the etiology.

Types:

1. **First degree** => P wave is followed by a QRS complex.
2. **Second degree, Mobitz I/Wenckebach** => progressive widening or lengthening of PR interval until a P wave is dropped.
3. **Second degree, Mobitz II** => P waves are blocked intermittently → QRS complexes are wide → PR interval is constant.
4. **Third degree** => no consistent pattern between the atrial and ventricle. The ventricular pattern has a wide QRS escape.

Lab Tests/Diagnostics:
1. Obtain an ECG, Echocardiography, cardiac enzymes, and electrolytes to determine any heart related etiology.
2. Check lyme serology for Lyme disease, TSH for hypothyroidism, or digoxin level for digoxin toxicity as the cause of heart block or Atrial Ventricular (AV) block.

Management:
1. Identify etiology and **discontinue** contributing medications.
2. Treat beta blocker or calcium channel blocker overdose with **glucagon**.
3. For calcium channel blocker overdose → treat with calcium chloride or calcium gluconate. Insulin and glucose may be required.
4. Unstable patients with hypotension and not responding to treatment as mentioned above should be treated with vasopressin.
5. Temporary or permanent pacemaker may be needed if drug therapy fails.

Aortic Dissection

- Symptoms => severe chest pain radiating to the back + long standing hypertension.
- Exam => look for aortic regurgitation.

Lab Tests/Diagnostics:
1. Chest x-ray shows **widened mediastinum** or an aortic knob.
2. Computed tomography (CT) scan with intravenous contrast is diagnostic.
3. Transesophageal echocardiography (TEE) is sensitive and specific.
4. Magnetic resonance imaging (MRI).
5. Affected **proximal arch or ascending aorta** need urgent surgery.

Treatment:
1. Start with beta blocker (esmolol), then with nitroprusside if there's difficulty controlling it and surgery is needed.
2. Urgent surgical repair with proximal arch or ascending aorta dissection. **THINK => Treat AAA with surgery if it is AA (Ascending Aorta).**

Complications:

- Observe for aortic rupture, cardiac tamponade, aortic regurgitation, and **limb or renal ischemia.**

- **Abdominal Aortic Aneurysm (AAA)** → screen/monitor with serial **ultrasound in smokers** and age > 65 if aneurysm is < 5cm. However, if aneurysm is ≥ 5cm, treat with surgery. If aneurysm is tender, plan an **urgent repair** (or if aneurysm is about 6cm in size) to avoid potential rupture. Any aneurysm causing chest pain that radiates to the back should be managed with **emergency surgery**.

PERIPHERAL VASCULAR DISEASE

1. Disease increases with risk factors such as advanced age, smoking, diabetes, hypertension, and hypercholesterolemia.
2. Smooth, shiny skin; may have loss of lower extremity pulses, loss of hair and sweat glands. If there's pain + pallor + loss of pulse => indicates occlusion in the artery.
3. PAD affects different organs such as the lower extremities, kidneys, mesenteric, and the brain.

Use history to differentiate pseudoclaudication from claudication:
- **Pseudoclaudication** pain occurs with **standing** → pain is relieved after **30 minutes** of **sitting**.
- **Claudication** pain occurs with **walking** → pain is relieved after **5 minutes** of **rest**.

Lab Tests/Diagnosis:

1. Lower extremities: Arterial-brachial index (**normal = > 0.9**), arterial Doppler (bruits), angiography, and MRA for revascularization if surgery is needed.
2. Kidneys: Doppler ultrasound, angiography, or MRA for renal artery stenosis.
3. Mesenteric ischemia: Angiography.

Treatment:

1. Lower extremities disease: Walking, cilostozol, pentoxyfilene, and clopidogrel (plavix).
2. Kidneys (renal artery disease): surgical revascularization or angioplasty.
3. Mesenteric ischemia: surgical revascularization or angioplasty.
4. Prevent or minimize risk factors by stopping smoking, controlling hypertension and diabetes. Start aspirin and statin.

HYPERCHOLESTEROLEMIA

1. Hypercholesterolemia increases the risk of arteriosclerosis.
2. Causes include: idiopathic, genetic, or secondary to diabetes, nephrotic syndrome, and hypothyroidism.
3. Findings => **xanthelasma**, **xanthomas** and **corneal arcus**.
4. Cholesterol-causing pancreatitis may indicate **familial hypertriglyceridemia**.
5. **Screen** asymptomatic patients without risk factors every 5 years by checking lipid panel.
6. A lipid panel consists of total cholesterol, high-density lipoprotein (HDL), low-density lipoprotein (LDL), and triglycerides. Low-density lipoprotein (LDL) and triglycerides are measured only when fasting.
7. High LDL and total cholesterol are risk factors for cardiovascular diseases. Either **LDL or total cholesterol** may be used in determining treatment.
8. Hypertriglyceridemia alone → not a risk factor for cardiovascular disease. However, when triglyceride level is > 500, treat with diet, exercise, and **gemfibrozil**.
9. Total cholesterol **> 300 => familial hypercholesterolemia.**
10. Check TSH and glucose.

Management:

1. Start with diet, exercise, and reduce smoking. Initiate medication if no response to lifestyle modification.
2. When a patient has cardiovascular diseases along with diabetes mellitus → target LDL < 70.
3. Treat hypercholesterolemia with → **statins, niacin**, or **cholestyramine (bile-acid binding resins)**; hypertriglyceridemia with → **gemfibrozil (fibrate)**; and low HDL (in order to increase) with → **niacin or fibrate**.
4. Check liver enzymes before initiating statins → look for side effect of muscle spasm.
5. Manage patients with diabetes.

HYPERTENSION

1. Defined as elevated blood pressure greater than 140/90 in two separate readings.
2. Primary hypertension is essentially hypertension only.
3. Secondary hypertension occurs before age 30 or after 55. Can be due to pheochromocytoma, hyperaldosteronism, hyperthyroidism, renal vascular hypertension, polycystic kidney disease, birth control pills, hypercalcemia, Cushing disease, Conn syndrome, coarctation of aorta, increased alcohol intake, and NSAIDs usage.

4. Findings => pheochromocytoma (**episodic hypertension**), hyperaldosteronism (**hypokalemia**), renal artery stenosis (**renal bruit**), and coarctation of aorta (**rib notching on chest x-ray**).
5. **Refractory hypertension** occurs when blood pressure cannot be controlled with **three or more** antihypertensive medications. Consider ruling out white coat hypertension, alcohol usage, volume overload, birth control pills, obstructive sleep apnea, and noncompliant patients.

Lab Tests/Diagnosis:

1. Primary hypertension is diagnosed **after two or more** separate measurements greater than 140/90.
2. Certain causes of secondary hypertension should be carefully evaluated before performing diagnostic tests.
3. Secondary hypertension may be diagnosed by checking PAC/PRA ratio > 20 and 24-hour urinary aldosterone (hyperaldosteronism), 24-hour urinary metanephrines or plasma metanephrines (pheochromocytoma), 24-hour urinary cortisol level or low-dose dexamethasone suppression test (Cushing disease), chest x-ray and MRA (coarctation of aorta), doppler ultrasound and renal artery MRA (renal artery stenosis), TSH (hyperthyroidism), and calcium (hypercalcemia).

Treatment:
1. Diuretics (thiazides) are first line of treatment in hypertension.
2. ACEI → for diabetic patients with nephropathy, microalbuminuria and congestive heart failure.
3. Beta blockers and ACEI should be considered in post MI patients to reduce risk of mortality.
4. Other antihypertensive medications are calcium channel blockers and hydralazine.
5. Renal artery stenosis → Diuretic +/- spironolactone, alpha blocker, hydralazine, or minoxidil. Revascularization with percutaneous transluminal angioplasty with stent.
6. Refractory hypertension → treated by adding nifedipine, hydralazine, minoxidil, or spironolactone.

HYPERTENSIVE URGENCY

1. Systolic blood pressure > 200 mmHg and/or diastolic blood pressure > 120 mmHg **without** any end-organ failure.
2. Patient may be asymptomatic.
3. Treat with **captopril**, **labetalol**, or **fenoldapam** (when beta blocker is contraindicated).

HYPERTENSIVE EMERGENCY

1. Systolic blood pressure > 200 mmHg and/or diastolic blood pressure > 120 mmHg **with** end-organ failure.
2. Patients may present with symptoms such as papilledema, encephalopathy, blindness, flash pulmonary edema, or congestive heart failure.
3. You may obtain arterial line to monitor mean arterial pressure (MAP).
4. Treat with **nitroprusside, labetalol, and nitroglycerin.**

PERICARDIAL DISEASE
PERICARDITIS

1. Inflammation of the pericardial sac may be due to idiopathic, viral, post MI (Dressler's syndrome), cancer, lupus, or tuberculosis.
2. There are 3 stages: **acute:** < 6 weeks; **subacute:** 6 weeks – 6 months; **chronic:** > 6 months.
3. Findings => **chest pain radiating to the back or shoulder (trapezius)** that is relieved with leaning forward or sitting up. Also listen for **friction rub** on examination.

Lab Tests/Diagnosis:

1. ECG → Be quick to observe for presence of diffuse ST-segment elevation and PR depression in V5-V6.
2. Echocardiography → check for pericardial effusion.
3. Elevated sedimentation rate (ESR).
4. Check for other causes by: blood cultures, ANA, and PPD.

Treatment:

1. Treat underlying disease.
2. NSAIDs (indomethacin, naprosyn, ibuprofen, or **aspirin**). Use aspirin in post MI patients to avoid complication with scar formation. Prednisone may be used only if pain persists after NSAIDs or aspirin trial.

Complications:

- Observe for pericardial effusion and cardiac tamponade.

PERICARDIAL EFFUSION AND CARDIAC TAMPONADE

1. Defined as the acute or chronic accumulation of fluid or blood in the pericardial cavity.
2. May be secondary to trauma.
3. **Findings** => elevated jugular venous pulse (JVP), distant or muffled heart sounds, pulsus paradoxus (on exam; decrease in blood pressure > 10 mm Hg on **inhalation**), electrical alternans (on EKG), and hypotension.
4. Other symptoms: shock and shortness of breath +/- chest pain, and heart failure.

Lab Tests/Diagnosis:

1. Chest x-ray (large cardiac silhouette).
2. ECG (low voltages & electrical alternans).
3. Echocardiography (most accurate; confirms fluid and diagnosis).
4. Right heart catheterization (equalization of all pressures in the heart during diastole).

Treatment:

- Pericardiocentesis (best initial); pericardial window placement (long-term).

CARDIOLOGY 1-LINER JUNKY CASES

- Vasovagal syncope → recommend 24-hour holter monitor.
- **Cocaine** → **worse with beta blocker** (due to unopposed blockade) → it causes HTN & ischemia.
- Myoglobin => is the **first to rise** after an MI chest pain out of all the cardiac enzymes.
- Status-post myocardial infarction, there's risk of reinfarction 5 days after → recheck cardiac enzyme (CK-MB).
- **Do not** perform stress test in acute cases → Note: stress test may be done when you are unable to find anything on ECG and enzyme labs.
- Status-post abnormal stress test that shows an area of only **reversible ischemia** in a patient without risk factors for CAD → order **angiography** as next diagnostic step for further management. If there is a **scar (indicates fixed defect)** → proceed with **angiogram first, then coronary artery bypass graft (CABG)**.
- Status-post balloon pump → place biventricular assist device → before you are able to perform heart transplant.
- Do **not** use nitroglycerin (nitrates) with sildenafil (Viagra) in post-MI patient having complaint of erectile dysfunction.
- AFib → shows irregular irregular QRS complex with **no P wave**.
- Stenosis > 70% in left main coronary artery + three coronary vessels with > 70% stenosis → **Tx/indications for CABG surgery**.
- Repair abdominal aortic aneurysm (AAA) → when size is > 5cm to prevent rupture.
- Status-post (AAA) repair → if there's bloody diarrhea → usually due to ischemic colitis → check proctosigmoidoscopy.
- Side effect: procainamide/hydralazine → lupus-like symptoms.
- Right-side heart failure → increased JVP, congested hepatomegaly, **peripheral edema**.
- Left-side heart failure → pulmonary edema (SOB, orthopnea, **cough**, paroxysmal nocturnal dyspnea).
- Indication for dual chambers → mobitz II second degree heart block, third-degree AV block, symptomatic bradycardia, and symptomatic hypertrophic cardiomyopathy with severe outlet obstruction.
- **Third-degree** heart block → **canon "a" waves**.
- Increased intracranial pressure → Tx: mannitol.
- Tricuspid atresia → decreased pulmonary vascular flow → blood can't flow from RA→RV.
- Transposition of great arteries → egg-shaped cardiac silhouette → increased pulmonary markings → Tx: Prostaglandin (PGE1).
- Hyperkalemia → EKG shows widened QRS complex → peaked T waves → Tx:

- calcium chloride or calcium gluconate.
- Small VSDs & muscular VSDs → close spontaneously.
- Tetralogy of Fallot → 'cry' or 'tet spells' → recommend repositioning with knees to chest to improve symptoms.
- Utero-cocaine exposure → complication => VSD.
- Normal wedge pressure => 11.
- Streptococcus bovis in infective endocarditis → due to GI cancer → check colonoscopy.
- Pulseless patients → first, emergency cardioversion → then, drug therapy.
- Unstable angina → ST segment depression in lateral leads V4-V6.
- Status-post unstable angina → check stress test 48-72 hours later.
- Hypertrophic cardiomyopathy & MVP → both have systolic murmurs which increase with valsalva maneuver.
- Aortic stenosis → mild situation: peaks early in systole → worse situation: peaks late in systole → @ 2nd right intercostal space.
- Aortic stenosis → due to congenital bicuspid aortic valve → if calcified → leads to outflow obstruction.
- No calcium channel blocker status-post acute ischemia!
- Turner syndrome (short stature, webbed neck, cubitus valgus) → risk of HTN → secondary to coarctation of aorta.
- Ectopic lentis → Marfan's syndrome.
- Aortic dissection → causes syncopal attack in Marfan's syndrome; while mitral valve prolapse → is usually asymptomatic.
- Anterior MI → ST elevation & Q waves in anterior leads V1, V2, & V3.
- Inferior MI → ST elevation & Q wave in inferior leads II, III, & AVF.
- **Aspirin => initial medication** for **all ischemic pain.**
- Decreased EF < 40% → increases mortality in post-MI.
- All patients scheduled for angioplasty & stent → should receive **clopidogrel.**
- Clopidogrel → given in acute MI, patients undergoing angioplasty, and in aspirin-allergy patients.
- Post-MI therapy/management which is **"time-dependent"** => **Aspirin, angioplasty, thrombolytics.**
- Angioplasty → given **< 90 mins** of onset of chest pain; Thrombolytics → given **90 mins to 12 hours** of onset of chest pain.
- Give thrombolytics → in cases of new LBBB status-post MI.
- Give **thrombolytics within 30 mins** of **ARRIVAL to ER.**
- Angioplasty lowers the risk of mortality status-post MI more than beta blocker.
- **Indications for thrombolytics → acute MI with ST segment elevation** shown **on ECG** (not dependent on cardiac enzymes) and **new LBBB status-post MI.**
- **Heparin, GPIIb/IIIa inhibitors** (tirofiban, eptifibatide, abciximab), and angioplasty are given → in non-ST segment elevation post-MI.
- **Echocardiography => initial test** to evaluate **valve dysfunction; Nuclear ventriculogram => most accurate** to evaluate **ejection fraction.**
- **Indication for statin therapy =>** Treatment for LDL > 130; CAD patients; and in **patients** with CAD equivalents (DM, PAD, aortic or carotid disease) with LDL

> 100.
- **LDL goal in CAD patients => < 100**.
- **LDL goal** in CAD + **diabetes** patients => **< 70**.
- Pulmonary edema **(acute)** => exacerbation of CHF & it is a **clinical diagnosis** →
  In ICU, treatment => oxygen + nitroglycerin + morphine + furosemide (by reducing preload). In patients **not** responding to treatment, **after 30 mins**, start positive inotropic agent such as **dobutamine**, amrinone, or milrinone. Other medications are spironolactone, atrial natriuretic peptide (ANP) and brain natriuretic peptide (BNP).
- You check **echocardiography** in acute pulmonary edema only **after stabilization of symptoms**.
- **Tx of ventricular tachycardia => lidocaine**; when **associated with acute pulmonary edema** → treat with **synchronized cardioversion**.
- Acute pulmonary edema + AFib, flutter, or supraventricular tachycardia => Tx: synchronized cardioversion.
- Persistent CHF with EF < 35% (despite tx for CHF) => manage with implantable cardioverter or defibrillator.
- Cardiogenic shock → diagnosis: Echocardiography + Swan-Ganz right heart catheterization → treatment: ACEIs + emergency revascularization.
- Right ventricular "infarction" → Right ventricular leads on ECG → manage with **IV fluids**.

Chapter 2
Endocrinology
Thyroid Disease

1. Initial screening is done with thyroid function tests: TSH, total T4, free T4, and free T3.
2. Antibody assay: includes anti-thyroid peroxidase (anti-TPO) antibodies, anti-microsomal antibodies, and thyroid stimulating immunoglobulins; and thyroid binding globulin.
3. Radiographic imaging: thyroid uptake scan => also known as radioactive iodine uptake scan (RAIU scan) and obtain a thyroid ultrasound.
4. Invasive testing: fine needle aspiration (FNA), thyroid biopsy, and surgery.

Hypothyroidism

1. **Causes**: Consider the following: Hashimoto thyroiditis, subacute thyroiditis, sick euthyroid syndrome, hypothyroidism from taking hyperthyroid medications, iatrogenic hypothyroidism due to thyroidectomy, and drug-induced hypothyroidism (such as lithium and amiodarone).
2. **Symptoms**: Look for: dry skin, coarse hair, fatigue, cold intolerance, constipation, bradycardia, weight gain, irregular menstruation, depression, decreased or slow deep tendon reflexes, dementia, hypercholesterolemia, myxedema, and arthralgias.
3. **Diagnosis**: start with TSH (high) and free thyroxine or T4 (low). Order further testing based upon symptoms and history. Low T4 and high TSH => **primary hypothyroidism**.
4. **Treatment**: thyroxine (T4).

Causes of hypothyroidism:

1. **Hashimoto thyroiditis**: this is an autoimmune disorder => most common cause of primary hypothyroidism → histology shows lymphocytic infiltration of the thyroid gland → painless thyroid enlargement → **diffuse** goiter → diagnose with anti-TPO antibodies or anti-microsomal antibodies → related to **pernicious anemia, vitiligo, lupus, addison's disease, and B-cell lymphoma** → treat with **levotyroxine**. Recheck TSH after 6 weeks of starting treatment.
2. **Subacute thyroiditis**: due to viral inflammation of the gland with symptoms of upper respiratory infection, fever, and tender thyroid gland → may be due to

mumps or coxsackievirus → diagnose with ESR (high), increased RAIU, and positive thyroglobulin antibody → treat with **NSAIDs or prednisone**; however patients can recover without treatment.

3. **Sick euthyroid syndrome:** seen in critically ill patients → there is usually a presence of an underlying illness → diagnosis is with TSH → condition is self-limiting.

4. **Lithium-induced hypothyroidism: patient becomes hypothyroid** after lithium use → do not discontinue lithium medication → **start levothyroxine** for hypothyroidism.

Complications:

Myxedema coma => it is a severe component of hypothyroidism that is due to untreated or under-treatment of hypothyroidism → presents with altered mental status, coma, and hypothermia → precipitated by underlying cause such as stress, trauma, or sepsis → treat first by stabilizing with mechanical ventilation, then use warming blankets, **IV levothyroxine, and IV hydrocortisone**. Also treat the underlying cause.

__Hyperthyroidism__

1. **Causes:** Consider the following: Grave's disease, toxic adenoma, toxic multi-nodular goiter, post-partum thyroiditis, and surreptious intake of thyroid hormones.

2. **Symptoms:** Look for: anxiety, tachycardia, sweaty skin, weight loss, heat intolerance, diarrhea, atrial fibrillation, oligomenorrhea or irregular menstruation, tremors, and osteoporosis.

3. **Diagnosis:** start with TSH (low) and free thyroxine or T4 (high). Order further testing based upon symptoms and history. High T4 and low TSH => **primary hyperthyroidism**.

4. **Treatment:** anti-thyroid drug propylthiouracil (PTU), thionamide (methimazole), radioactive 131I thyroid ablation, **beta blocker (propanolol) for symptomatic** hyperthyroidism, and surgery (thyroidectomy).

Causes of hyperthyroidism:

1. **Grave's disease**: this occurs due to an antibody at TSH receptor → **diffuse, non-tender** goiter → exophthalmos, proptosis, lid lag, diplopia, pretibial myxedema → **thyroid bruit or thrill** → diagnose with low TSH, high T4, **increased** RAIU, positive thyroid-stimulating immunoglobulin, and thyroglobulin antibody → treat with propylthiouracil or methimazole first, then with 131I thyroid ablation, and surgery (thyroidectomy). Propranolol is used to treat tremors and palpitations.

2. **Toxic adenoma: increased** RAIU at location of palpable nodule.

3. **Toxic multi-nodular goiter:** several nodules on goiter → treatment: surgery.

4. **Amiodarone-induced thyrotoxicosis:** Type 1: related to **goiter and iodine overload** → treat with methimazole +/- potassium perchlorate. Type 2: related to **drug-induced follicular damage thyroiditis** → treat with corticosteroids → if resistant to treatment, treat with dialysis, plasmapheresis, or thyroidectomy.

Evaluation of thyroid nodule: Start with TSH.

1. Low TSH => Hyperthyroidism → check RAIU scan → if increased (hot nodule), treat with 131I ablation therapy and follow up. If decreased (cold nodule), check fine needle aspiration (FNA).
2. High TSH => Hypothyroidism → check thyroid ultrasound → if suspicious, check FNA → if ultrasound is normal, proceed with checking free T4, anti-TPO antibodies, and anti-microsomal antibodies. Treat.
3. Indication for FNA => nodule **> 10mm** in size and **suspicious** thyroid on ultrasound.

Therapy and Side Effects:
1. **PTU** (rash, agranulocytosis, and hepatocellular necrosis) → preferred in pregnancy & breast feeding → discontinue PTU and check CBC after complaints of rash, fever, and sore throat. Initial follow up to check TSH level should be done within 6-8 weeks of initiating therapy.
2. **Methimazole** → Can cause rash, agranulocytosis, and cholestatic jaundice. It is also the cause of **aplasia cutis:** absence of skin on scalp of newborns.
3. **Radioiodine therapy** → treatment measurement depends on goiter size and RAIU scan → avoid in pregnancy & breast feeding → avoid in Grave's ophthalmopathy → may use radioiodine therapy with corticosteroid → avoid contact with children after radioiodine treatment → risk of hypothyroidism with radioiodine treatment: check TSH and treat with levothyroxine.
4. **Surgery:** indications => multi-nodular goiter, large goiter with obstructive symptoms (Plummer disease; do total lobectomy), recurrence of goiter, non-compliance, cancer, and pregnancy → **prior to surgery**, make **euthyroid**: first with methimazole, iodine per oral, then total thyroidectomy. Status-post surgery, there is risk of recurrent laryngeal nerve palsy, hypoparathyroidism, and hypocalcemia (replace with calcium to prevent spasms).

Complications: Thyroid storm => severe hyperthyroidism → significant for fever, tachycardia, dehydration, and coma → treatment is with iodine, propylthiouracil or methimazole, dexamethasone, and propranolol.

Adrenal Insufficiency

1. **Primary adrenal insufficiency** (Addison's disease) => adrenal failure and autoimmune (idiopathic) is the most common cause (**low ACTH**). Addison

disease => **loss of aldosterone**. Other causes are due to hemorrhagic infarction and malignancy.

2. **Secondary adrenal insufficiency** => as a result of previous use of exogenous steroids (**high ACTH**) → usually presents during surgery with **hypotension and electrolyte imbalance**.

3. **Other causes: Sheehan syndrome** (pituitary infarction with patient not able to breast feed post-partum) and pituitary tumor.

4. Symptoms: are precipitated by stress, trauma, or surgery → presents with **increased hyperpigmentation of skin ('tanned')**, fatigue, weight loss, nausea, vomiting, abdominal pain, anorexia, diarrhea, hypotension, syncope, and shock.

5. **Diagnosis**: Check serum A.M. cortisol, **ACTH stimulation test (cosyntropin stimulation test)**, hyponatremia, hyperkalemia, and eosinophilia. **CT scan of the adrenal gland.**

6. **Treatment**: Fluids + Hydrocortisone + Mineralocorticoids. Prednisone may be given to stable patients without hypotension. **Fludrocortisone** may be added in cases of hypotension, hyponatremia, and hyperkalemia.

Complications:

Addisonian crisis => includes the symptoms of adrenal insufficiency + confusion + shock → treat crisis with supportive management including IV fluids and IV hydrocortisone.

Cushing's Syndrome

1. Etiologies: adrenal (adenoma), pituitary (adenoma), ectopic (small cell carcinoma of the lung), and exogenous use.

2. Symptoms: Carefully observe for moon faces, "buffalo hump," truncal obesity, easy bruising and abdominal striae, hypertension, muscle weakness, amenorrhea, hiruitism, impotence, and neurological disturbances (depression and psychosis).

3. Diagnosis: 1 mg low-dose dexamethasone suppression test, **24-hour urinary cortisol (increased, best initial test)**, A.M. stimulation test (ACTH), high-dose dexamethasone suppression test → CT scan (**adrenal adenoma**); obtain a MRI to rule out ACTH-secreting **pituitary adenoma** and Ectopic ACTH-producing tumors such as carcinoid tumors or small cell lung cancer.

4. Treatment: consider surgical removal.

Pheochromocytoma

1. Severe intermittent or episodic hypertension + headaches + orthostatic hypotension + tremors + palpitations + dizziness + diaphoresis. Associated with

multiple endocrine neoplasia (MEN) type IIa syndrome along with medullary thyroid cancer and parathyroid hyperplasia.

2. Diagnosis: Initially, **obtain 24-hour urine metanephrines (most specific)**, catecholamines, or vanillylmandelic acid (VMA). If positive, obtain **CT scan of the abdomen to confirm adrenal mass or MRI**. Obtain metaiodobenzylguanidine (MIBG) scan only to rule out metastasis or extra adrenal masses.

3. Treatment: Initially, use phentholamine IV or nitroprusside → alpha and beta adrenergic blockers (**phenoxybenzamine + atenolol**) prior to surgery → consider surgery or laparoscopic resection of tumor.

Hyperprolactinemia: Prolactinoma

1. Functional pituitary tumor → hyperprolactinemia.
2. Prolactin inhibits GnRH @ pituitary → decreased LH, FSH, and testosterone.
3. Hyperprolactinemia may also be due to drugs such as phenothiazines, metoclopromide, or tricyclic antidepressants (TCAs). Other causes of hyperprolactinemia => nipple stimulation + pregnancy + stress + exercise + hypothyroidism + depression + chest wall irritation.
4. Symptoms: galactorrhea, amenorrhea, headaches, diplopia, and temporary visual field loss. **Men** may have impotence, gynecomastia, and decreased libido.
5. Diagnosis: Obtain prolactin level (**increased**) → if < 100 => due to stress, drugs, or pregnancy. If > 100-500 => due to prolactinoma (microadenoma, < 3mm). If > 500-1000 => due to macroadenoma with symptoms related to mass effect. May obtain **LH and FSH** levels (**both decreased**). Obtain an MRI to confirm location of pituitary tumor.
6. Treatment: manage stress properly, discontinue drugs; use dopamine agonists such as **bromocriptine** and cabergoline. Surgery (transsphenoidal) +/- irradiation if tumor is large or medical therapy is not tolerated.
7. For accidentally-found pituitary adenomas on a CT scan, **check functionality first** by obtaining ACTH, TSH, or prolactin levels.
8. Rule out pregnancy first in all reproductive females. Rule out drugs and stress.

Conn's Syndrome

1. Aldosterone-producing tumor (adrenal adenoma).
2. Diagnosis: aldosterone (high), hypertension, hypokalemia, alkalosis, low renin, and **PAC/PRA ratio**. If positive results, obtain **CT scan of abdomen** (confirms and to rule out adrenal tumor).
3. **Hypokalemia** may result in **motor weakness** and **nephrogenic diabetes insipidus** (polyuria + polydipsia).

4. Treatment: **Spironolactone** initially, and surgery if tumor > 4cm or medical therapy is not tolerated.

For **accidentally-found adrenal adenomas** on a CT scan, **check functionality first** by obtaining low-dose dexamethasone suppression test and plasma metanephrines. If functioning, surgery is recommended. If non-functioning and tumor size is < 4cm, follow-up with CT scan at 6 months. If > 4-6cm, follow-up with CT scan at 6 months or perform surgery. If > 6cm, perform surgery (more risk of cancer).

Insulinoma

1. Beta cell tumor type.
2. Symptoms: Whipple's triad: hypoglycemia + CNS symptoms (confusion and loss of consciousness). Symptoms onset is usually after fasting.
3. Diagnosis: **Hypoglycemia + hyperinsulinemia + C-peptide level (increased) + proinsulin level (increased).**
4. Treatment: Immediate relief with glucose (e.g. by eating a granola bar) and resection of tumor.

Surreptitious insulin use: Hypoglycemia + hyperinsulinemia + **C-peptide level (decreased) + proinsulin level (decreased).**

Glucagonoma

1. Alpha cell tumor type → islet of Langherhan's.
2. Consider it: Hyperglycemia + migratory necrotizing skin erythema.
3. Diagnosis: Octreotide scan, plasma glucagon levels, CT abdomen, arteriography, and somatostatin receptor scintigraphy (SRS).
4. Treatment: Octreotide (somastostatin). Oral zinc for dermatitis.
5. Metastases at time of diagnosis → treat with chemo: streptozotocin and dacarbazine.
6. Complications: Diabetes → venous thrombosis → pulmonary embolus.

Primary Hyperparathyroidism

1. This is an adenoma.
2. Symptoms: Be on a lookout for constipation + nausea + fatigue + bone pain + polyuria + polydipsia + confusion. Presents with symptoms of **hypercalcemia.**

3. Diagnosis: Hypercalcemia + high PTH + low PO4.
4. Treatment: **Parathyroidectomy** (surgery). **Hydrate with IV fluids** + diuretic (furosemide) **after** volume deficit is corrected. **Bisphosphonate** (alendronate or pamidronate) for **chronic therapy** of <u>severe</u> hypercalcemia **> 14 mg/dL** (usually with **underlying cancer**).
5. May be associated with multiple endocrine neoplasia (MEN) syndrome.

- **Indications for Parathyroidectomy (Surgery): Hypercalcemia** > 12 mg/dL, hypercalciuria or urinary calcium excretion > 400 mg/day, nephrolithiasis, osteitis fibrosa cystica, kidney failure, age < 50, osteoporosis, pregnancy, and neurological problems such as delirium, depression, confusion, or psychosis.
- **Risk of hypocalcemia with surgery** → symptoms include seizures + muscle cramps or twitching of nerves **(Chvostek's sign)** + **hungry bone syndrome** (after parathyroid adenoma removal) + recurrent laryngeal nerve palsy + prolonged QT seen on ECG. Treat with calcium +/- vitamin D.
- **Hypocalcemia** → causes are due to parathyroidectomy, vitamin D deficiency, PTH resistance, fat malabsorption, and hyperphosphatemia.

Diabetes Mellitus

Type I Diabetes Mellitus:

1. Insulin deficiency due to destruction of pancreatic beta cells → autoimmune.
2. Symptoms: Consider looking for polyphagia + polydipsia + polyuria + blurry vision + weight loss + infections-prone such as candidiasis and some bacteria.
3. Diagnosis: Get two sets of: Fasting plasma glucose ≥ 126 mg/dL, or random glucose ≥ 200 mg/dL, or two-postprandial glucose of ≥ 200 mg/dL after a 75-g oral glucose load, and you have a diagnosis.
4. Related to HLA DR3 and DR4. Risk of **diabetic ketoacidosis (DKA)**.
5. Treatment: **Insulin** (basal and bolus) or with multi-daily injection (MDI) regimen.

Diabetic Ketoacidosis: Complication of type I diabetes with precipitation due to stressors such as infection, sepsis, surgery, or noncompliance → patient presents with hyperglycemia, metabolic acidosis (**low bicarbonate**), and ketonuria. **Serum bicarbonate** determines **severity. Low bicarbonate => increased anion gap.** Also beta hydroxybutyrate => ketone marker. Decreased levels of beta hydroxybutyrate => positive indication of ketones resolved. DKA patient will **hyperventilate** to compensate for metabolic acidosis.

Lab Tests/Diagnosis:

- Obtain glucose, complete blood count (CBC), ABG, BUN/creatinine, serum ketones, serum osmolality, chemistry, urine analysis, urine and blood cultures, and ECG.

Treatment:

1. Administer fluids (normal saline, NS) and IV regular insulin.
2. Monitor glucose level, potassium, phosphate, sodium, and ABG with anion gap every two hours. Replace potassium and phosphate.
3. When glucose < 250 mg/L, **change** NS to D5NS.
4. When anion gap becomes normal, **change** IV regular insulin to subcutaneous insulin sliding scale.

Complication: cerebral edema (treat with mannitol).

Type II Diabetes Mellitus:

1. Due to increased insulin resistance.
2. Symptoms: Consider looking for polyphagia + polydipsia + polyuria + blurry vision +/- weight loss + infection(s)-prone such as candidiasis.
3. Diagnosis: fasting plasma glucose $\geq$ 126 mg/dL, or random glucose $\geq$ 200 mg/dL, or two-postprandial glucose of $\geq$ 200 mg/dL after a 75-g oral glucose load. (Same as Type I).
4. Treatment: Recommend a healthy diet low in fat and carbohydrate. Start oral hypoglycemic medications such as a glitazone (metformin), sulfonylurea (glyburide). Add/start insulin (NPH or glargine) with difficult-to-control hyperglycemia.

Hyperglycemic Hyperosmolar Nonketotic State (HHNK): Complication of type II diabetes mellitus precipitated by infection, dehydration, and drugs. Administer fluids (normal saline, NS) and give IV regular insulin only if hyperglycemia persists after fluid resuscitation. Monitor glucose level, potassium, phosphate, sodium, and ABG. Replace potassium and phosphate. Treat the precipitating factor.

Health Maintenance & Complications:

1. Obtain hemoglobin A1c (HbA1c) level which should be maintained < 6.5.
2. Blood pressure management in type II DM => < 130/80.
3. **Nephropathy:** Follow-up annually to monitor renal disease by checking **urine microalbumin**. Start **ACEIs** for patients with diabetic nephropathy even with normal BP.
4. **Neuropathy:** Perform a foot exam annually for neuropathy, ulcers, and peripheral vascular disease. Strict glycemic helps to control nerve conduction. Treat with **gabapentin or pregabalin** first, or with tricyclic antidepressants, and carbamazepine.
5. Recommend a healthy diet low in fat and carbohydrate or refer to nutritionist.

6. Obtain an ECG for patients > 35 years old or with underlying heart disease.
7. **Retinopathy:** Refer to ophthalmologist annually for evaluation of vision.
8. Screen and manage risk factors for heart disease such as hypertension, cholesterol, and smoking.
9. **Gastroparesis:** impaired motility in chronic DM→ symptoms of bloating, constipation and diarrhea → diagnose with gastric emptying scan → treat with metoclopromide or erythromycin.

ENDOCRINOLOGY 1-LINER JUNKY CASES

- **Metformin** → inhibits gluconeogenesis → best to use for **obese patients** → decreases weight gain → causes lactic acidosis → no risk of hypoglycemia. Do not use in renal failure or with contrast agents.
- Sulfonylurea (glyburide) → increases insulin release → increases weight gain; risk of hypoglycemia & **SIADH**.
- Silent thyroiditis → autoimmune, non-tender gland with hyperthyroidism → **normal RAIU** → no treatment needed.
- Goiter → not direct indicative of type of thyroid disease → need further observation and labs before diagnosis.
- **Calcitonin** → used to treat hypercalcemia when hydration and furosemide have failed to work → works faster than bisphosphonate → bisphosphonate takes weeks to work.
- **Steroid** → used to treat hypercalcemia in granulomatous diseases, vitamin D toxicity, and malignancy.
- **Exogenous Abuse of Thyroid Hormone** → "atrophy" of thyroid gland.
- Low ACTH => in adrenal gland → check with CT scan/MRI (e.g. adenoma).
- High ACTH => in pituitary gland or ectopic production of ACTH → check with CT scan/MRI (e.g. small cell cancer of the lung or carcinoid tumor).
- **Kallman's Syndrome** => **anosmia** + hypogonadism + delayed puberty + amenorrhea → in **hypothalamus** with **decreased** GnRH, LH, FSH, and estradiol.
- Increased cortisol + increased ACTH with high-dose suppression test + if MRI shows no abnormality or it is indeterminant → check **petrosal venous sinus sampling** → helps to localize lesion, then surgery.
- **Congenital adrenal hyperplasia (CAH)** → diagnosis: increased ACTH + increased testosterone + decreased cortisol + decreased aldosterone → treat with cortisol + aldosterone.
- **CAH** may also have hypoglycemia → due to cortisol deficiency.
- Watch for patients with CAH who will present with salt-wasting (hyponatremia), hyperkalemia, ambiguous genitalia, and skin pigmentation (genitalia) → it is due to **21-hydroxylase deficiency**.
- **Acromegaly** => in pituitary → increased release of growth hormone (GH) from GH secreting adenoma → findings include enlarged head, fingers, feet, jaw, and nose, amenorrhea, hypertension, sweating, cardiomegaly, and abnormal joints → risk of **diabetes** and **colonic polyps** → diagnose with insulin-like growth factor (IGF) (**best initial and confirms**), GH suppression by giving glucose, and MRI for pituitary adenoma → treat with bromocriptine/carbegoline, octreotide (somatostatin), GH receptor antagonist, or surgical removal (transphenoidal).
- **Turner Syndrome** => **also associated** with coarctation of aorta + delayed puberty + amenorrhea + hyperglycemia + hypothyroidism + cardiac & renal anomalies + GH resistance → can treat with GH.

- **Klinefelter's Syndrome** => 47 XXY → insensitivity of FSH and LH receptors on testicles → hypogonadism + amenorrhea + breasts **without cervix** or ovaries + blind pouch at vagina + mental retardation + wide hips + **small testes** → diagnose with **increased FSH, LH**, and **no testosterone** → treat with testosterone.
- **Diabetes Insipidus** => deficiency or unresponsiveness of antidiuretic hormone (ADH) → hyponatremia + loss of consciousness + confusion after head injury + polydipsia + polyuria.
- Hypothyroidism and depression → can cause hyperprolactinemia.
- Cushing Syndrome → easy bruising & striae => due to decreased collagen from cortisol by causing thinning of the skin.
- Hypertension in Cushing Syndrome => due to fluid & sodium retention.
- VIPoma => elevated VIP levels + profuse watery diarrhea → leads to **hypokalemia**.
- Polycystic ovarian syndrome (PCOS) => amenorrhea/oligomenorrhea + anovulation + hirsutism → diagnosis: increased testosterone, increased LH/FSH ratio, increased dehydroepiandrosterone sulfate (DHEAS), and increased glucose.
- Congenital hypothyroidism => feeding intolerance + **large tongue**.
- Familial hypocalciuric hypercalcemia => positive family history of hypercalcemia + patient with hypercalcemia + decreased urinary calcium excretion + increased PTH + decreased serum phosphate.

Chapter 3
Dermatology
<u>Vitiligo</u>

1. Autoimmune → antibodies to melanin → leads to depigmentation.
2. Consider looking for association with other autoimmune diseases such as pernicious anemia, addison's disease, and hypothyroidism (Hashimoto thyroiditis).
3. Diagnosis: clinical.
4. Treatment: may consider starting with topical corticosteroid (betamethasone), then with calcipotriol, and immunomodulator (tacrolimus) for < 20% or smaller parts of the body. For larger affected areas, use **monobenzone** for depigmentation, or **laser repigmentation** if no response.

<u>Tinea Vesicolor</u>

1. Caused by *Pityrosporum* infection.
2. Multiple hyper and hypo-pigmented scaly patches on the trunk that **fails to tan** for months even after treatment → appear as **'white spots' but may be brown or dark too.** Mostly apparent during **summer** due to inability to tan.
3. Diagnosis: Potassium hydroxide (KOH) mount preparation of lesion (hyphae and yeast) and wood's lamp (pale yellow fluorescence).
4. Treatment: Topical selenium sulfide lotion (and shampoo) and ketaconazole cream. Systemic symptoms are treated with oral ketoconazole, itraconazole, or fluconazole.

Fungal Infection of the feet, skin, and scalp:
1. Tinea corporis: Affects body or torso → red, ring-shaped lesions.
2. Tinea pedis: Affects foot (athlete's foot) → itching, web spaces between toes, and thick and disfigured toenails (onychomycosis).
3. Tinea capitis: Scaly patches of hair loss mostly on children → very contagious → presents with kerion (tender granuloma of scalp).
4. Tinea cruris: Affects crural folds of the thighs (jock itch) → mostly obese males.
5. **Diagnosis**: All with KOH preparation by scraping lesions and wood's lamp. Positive fluorescence of hair in tinea capitis indicates Microsporum etiology; otherwise, it's Trichophyton. Also **culture of the fungus** (most accurate).
6. **Treatment**: Mild cases are treated with topical antifungals such as topical

> ketoconazole—risk of hepatoxicity + gynecomastia). Tinea capitis and onychomycosis are treated with oral antifungals such as itraconazole, **terbinafine**—risk of hepatoxicity (check LFTs), or fluconazole.

Psoriasis

1. Signs and Symptoms: Be sure to look for: arthritis (**DIP joint**), **sausage-shaped fingers,** pitting of nails and onycholysis, **silvery, scaling papules and plaques** behind the ears, scalps, and extensor surfaces of the elbows and knees.
2. **Guttate psoriasis**: affects the **trunk**. May be treated with **phototherapy**.
3. **Erythrodermic psoriasis**: erythematous, scaling and exfoliation of the skin → **medical emergency**.
4. Diagnosis: clinical or biopsy if diagnosis is questionable. **Rheumatoid factor-negative**.
5. Treatment: For localized lesions, use topical corticosteroids, anthralin, tar (coal) preparations, **mineral oil**, vitamin D (**calcipotriene**) and vitamin A (topical **tazarotene**) analogs have all been used. Other: salicylic acid has been considered in management as well. For generalized lesions, anything more than 30% of the body, use **phototherapy**. Treat psoriasis arthritis with NSAIDs initially; then consider methotrexate or etanercept for more advanced disease.

Scabies

1. Caused by *Sarcoptes scabei* (mite).
2. Check out the burrows with lesions (wavy, threadlike and grayish-white) in **finger web spaces**, axilla, flexor surface of wrist, buttocks, and areola.
3. Patients complain of severe itching and pruritus → may cause **secondary bacterial infection**.
4. Diagnosis: scrape the lesions within the burrow after application of mineral oil → look under microscope for mites → skin biopsy (confirms diagnosis).
5. Treatment: **Permethrin** cream, lindane, topical malathion, or ivermectin. Permethrin is preferred over lindane (causes neurotoxicity).
6. Treat **all** members of family and close contacts even if asymptomatic. High rate of recurrence.

THINK: L. I. M. P. => Lindane → Ivermectin → Malathion → Permethrin (first).

Lice

1. Also known as pediculosis → affects the head *(Pediculus capitis)*, body *(Pediculus corporis)*, and pubic area *(Phthirus pubis)*.
2. Look for a patient complaining of severe itching at the pubic area → sexually transmitted.
3. Diagnosis: with magnification, observe lice on hair shafts.
4. Treatment: Permethrin cream.

Remember to : Change, wash, sterilize/boil bed sheets and other forms of clothing.

Lichen Planus

1. White, lacy striae and patches of white lines and dots lesions on the mouth.
2. The 4 P's: **p**ruritic, **p**urple, **p**olygonal **p**apules on wrists or ankles.
3. Diagnosis: clinical or biopsy (lichenoid lesions).
4. Treatment: self-limiting or topical corticosteroids (if erosion and pain exist). Symptom such as pruritus may be relieved with antihistamines.

Acne Vulgaris

- Comedones, papules, pustules, nodules, and cysts.
- **Treatment of Mild to Moderate** acne: **Comedonal → start with topical benzoyl peroxide gel →** if treatment fails, discontinue benzoyl peroxide gel and use **topical tretinoin acid** (comedolytic) **+/- topical erythromycin or clindamycin**.
- **Treatment of Moderate to Severe** acne: **Nodular + Pustular + Cystic → ADD** oral antibiotics (tetracycline, erythromycin, doxycycline, or TMP-SMX) to the treatment of moderate acne (above). You may also consider spironolactone.
- Decrease the androgenic effects in oral contraceptive pills (OCPs) if worsening acne → use third-generation OCPs. May add spironolactone (antiandrogenic) for severe acne.
- Isotretinoin → used for **severe acne** → you must monitor beta HCG→ need two forms of contraception before use → because it is very teratogenic → Also monitor side effects: liver function tests (high) and triglycerides (high). Other side effects of isotretinoin are dry skin, peeling of palms and soles, intracranial hypertension, and night blindness.

Rosacea

1. Similar to acne, which usually affect mostly adolescents and teenagers, rosacea affects mostly adults → present in middle age 40-50 years old.
2. Findings: Consider looking for erythema, pustules, papules, talengiectasis, facial flushing, **no comedones**, and **rhinophyma** is common (**hypertrophy of connective tissue and sebaceous gland hyperplasia**).
3. Worse with alcohol, sun exposure, hot climate/temperature, hot drinks, spicy foods, and emotional stress.
4. Diagnosis: clinical.
5. Treatment: Start with **topical metronidazole or azaleic acid**. For **persistent symptoms** and **ocular problems** such as blepharitis and keratitis, **use oral antibiotics** (tetracycline, minocycline) for a month then taper.
6. For **rhinophyma**, use **oral antibiotics first, then surgery** if no response to treatment.
7. Refractory cases: use topical metronidazole or retinoic acid.
8. Preventive measures: Consider educating patients to reduce stressors, avoid hot drinks, sun exposure or spicy foods.
9. May add clonidine or propranolol to relieve symptom of flushing.

Atopic Dermatitis (Eczema)

1. They appear as dry lichenified plaques that are pruritic and found on the neck, wrists, neck, and trunk.
2. Personal and family history of allergies, atopy, or asthma may be present. May also present in childhood with plaque eruptions in diaper area.
3. Risk of bacterial infection due to skin breaks from scratching.
4. Diagnosis: Clinical; obtain serum IgE (increased).
5. Treatment: Emmollient use by keeping skin moistened → use antihistamines and topical steroid creams (taper off) → may also use tacrolimus (steroid-sparing). Topical **doxepin** may be used for pruiritus.

Contact Dermatitis

1. Skin inflammation is caused by exposure to allergens or offending agents (poison ivy or nickel).
2. Type IV hypersensitivity reaction occurs with exposure to allergens.
3. Findings: look out for pruritic rash, itching, and burning.
4. Diagnosis: Usually **clinical**; detailed history is key → **patch testing** may also be

done (definitive test).

5. Treatment: Ideally, **avoid offending agent** → soothing preparations like oatmeal baths, cold compresses, and antihistamines (diphenhydramine) → **topical steroids (triamcinolone) or oral steroids** (for larger affected areas of the body).

Erythema Nodosum

1. Think of idiopathic process involving inflammation of skin and subcutaneous tissue → **painful**, red or violet nodules over the pretibial (shins).
2. May also be due to sarcoidosis (**good prognosis**), ulcerative colitis (**bad prognosis**), coccidiomycosis, pregnancy, histoplasmosis, syphilis, streptococcal infection, *Yersinia* infection, or tuberculosis.
3. Findings: fever, fatigue, tender lesions, athralgia, recent upper respiratory infection, or diarrhea.
4. Treatment: Self-limiting → NSAIDs for arthritic pain → potassium iodide drops and corticosteroids are helpful.

Erythema Multiforme

1. Etiology: drugs (penicillamine, NSAIDs, phenytoin, sulfa), infections (Herpes Simplex virus and *Mycoplasma*), pregnancy, connective tissue disorder, radiotherapy, and cancers.
2. **Target lesions (non-tender)** and papules on the **palms** and **soles** → **may recur.**
3. May present in severe form as **Stevens Johnson syndrome** → treat supportively.
4. Diagnosis: Usually clinical; however, biopsy may also be done.
5. Treatment: Provide symptoms relief with antihistamines. Treat the etiology.

- **Stevens Johnson syndrome**: affects the mucous membranes (oral mucosa, **respiratory tract**, and eye) → treat patients with respiratory problems in a **designated burn center**.

Pemphigus Vulgaris

1. Autoimmune disease → autoantibodies that cause destruction of intracellular adhesions that are located between skin's epithelial cells. May be caused by drugs (penicillamine, ACEIs); however, they are usually idiopathic. Skin destroys because they are so 'thin'.
2. Findings: **painful, flaccid bullae** from the **oral mucosa** and spreads to the body.

Esophagus may be affected. Also look for **nikolsky's sign** (skin peels easily).
3. Diagnosis: **skin biopsy** stained for antibody (shows **lacelike immunofluorescence pattern**).
4. Treatment: corticosteroids first, then azathiaprine/mycophenolate.

Pemphigus Pemphigoid

1. Autoimmune disease → autoantibodies that attack the basement membrane of the skin.
2. Findings: **subepidermal bullae** → large, tense bullae. Skin lesions here are thicker than pemphigus vulgaris; so pemphigus pemphigoid is less serious.
3. Diagnosis: Skin biopsy stained for antibody (shows **linear immunofluorescence pattern**).
4. Treatment: corticosteroids first, then erythromycin.

Herpes Zoster

- Etiology: reactivation of varicella-zoster virus.
- Findings: **painful** vesicles that change to crusted lesions in a **dermatomal distribution**.
- Diagnosis: clinical, but you may obtain tzanck smear (**giant cells**).
- Treatment: Acyclovir or valacyclovir. If started within 72 hours of onset, it can help to **decrease duration and occurrence** of post-herpetic neuralgia. Other medications include **gabapentin** (for post-herpetic neuralgia), topical capsaicin, and antidepressants (TCAs). Remember to vaccinate nonimmunized patients within 96 hours of exposure for chicken pox.
- Herpes zoster carries the risk of post-herpetic neuralgia.

Actinic Keratoses

1. Sun exposed area leading to **premalignant lesions for squamous cell carcinoma.**
2. Flesh colored, red papules.
3. Diagnosis: biopsy of lesion. Squamous cell carcinoma **in situ => Bowen disease.**
4. Treatment: If biopsy is suspicious, perform **excision of lesion. Cryotherapy, imiquimod**, or **curettage** can be used for treatment. **5-flourouracil** may be used if there are many lesions. Sunscreen also helps to reduce recurrences.

Seborrheic Keratoses

1. Appears on elderly as 'stuck-on' lesions.
2. Benign lesions → yellowish-waxy plaques or hyperpigmented lesions on the skin that may appear anywhere from the face, shoulder, and to the back.
3. Treatment: liquid nitrogen and curettage.

Basal Cell Carcinoma

1. Pink pearly papule. Involves sun exposure.
2. Diagnosis: Biopsy of lesion (confirms; punch or shave biopsy).
3. Treatment: **MOHs micrographic surgery**.

Malignant Melanoma

1. Superficial spreading melanoma => most common type of melanoma (70%) → better prognosis than nodular melanoma (vertically spread = depth). **Prognosis is based on depth.**
2. Risk factors: family history of melanoma, fair skin, history of severe sunburn with sun exposure, and multiple dysplastic nevi syndrome.
3. Look for signs of high-risk, skin carcinoma: **A**symmetry, **B**order (irregular), **C**olor (dark/variations), **D**iameter (> 6mm), **E**levation with surface irregularity.
4. Diagnosis: Biopsy of the skin.
5. Treatment: Surgery (surgical excision of the skin lesion) and chemotherapy. Use **interferon** to reduce recurrences.

DERMATOLOGY 1-LINER JUNKY CASES

- Alopecia areata => autoimmune → patches of hair loss → diagnose with KOH preparation of scraping, TSH, ESR, ANA, PPD, RPR, CBC → treat with intralesional triamcinolone +/- minoxidil or topical corticosteroid (kenalog).

- Side effects of topical corticosteroids => skin atrophy, striae, steroid acne, and rebound papular dermatitis.

- Stasis dermatitis => due to **venous insufficiency** of the lower extremities that is **irreversible** → **hemosiderin** deposited in the tissue causes **hyperpigmentation** → treatment: elevation of the lower extremities and support hose.

- **Porphyria Cutanea Tarda** => genetic predisposition → defective enzyme uroporphyrinogen decarboxylase → increase in porphyrins in liver → due to estrogens (OCPs), alcohol, liver disease, iron overload, or blood disorder such as thalasemia → dark urine, sensitive to sun (**photosensitivity reaction**), skin hyperpigmentation, and hypertrichosis of the face → associated with hepatitis C → diagnosis: increased urine porphyrins and positive fluorescence on wood's lamp → treatment: use sun tanning creams, avoid alcohol, discontinue estrogens, **therapeutic phleobotomy** (for iron overload), then **deferoxamine**, and **chloroquine** (alternative for iron overload or in milder cases).

- **Angioedema** => swelling of skin and mucous membrane which can lead to life-threatening airway edema → acquired or hereditary (autosomal dominant; due to C1 esterase Inhibitor deficiency) → diagnosis: **measure complement components (decreased C2 and C4)** → treat with danazol, C1 esterase Inhibitor, or fresh frozen plasma.

- Discontinue ACEIs and ARBs causing angioedema. If laryngeal edema is present with stridor → intubate.

- Molluscum contagiosum => *poxvirus* infection → lesions have inclusion bodies → treat with **freezing or curettage**.

- Bacillus Anthracis (**anthrax**) => in soil with spores; contact is from infected livestock → red pustule painless lesion on arm → evolved to thick black scab (black eschar with vesicles) → diagnose with **gram stain** (confirms) = **gram (+) bacilli** → treat with antibiotics (ciprofloxacin, penicillin, doxycycline) → associated with postal workers, wool sorters, and bioterrorism.

- **Kaposi Sarcoma** => due to Human *Herpes* virus 8 → patients with AIDS CD4 <

100 → **purple** skin lesions including oral mucosal → hint: **does not respond to multiple treatments** → treatment: initiate **HAART therapy** (increases CD4 levels) or **chemotherapy** (vinblastine + adriamycin) if HAART fails.

- Leukoplakia => white-colored plaque → **benign** oral lesion due to smoking and drinking alcohol → usually resolves with alcohol and smoking cessation.

- Hairy leukoplakia => EBV → oral lesions found in HIV patients.

- Lyme disease => diagnosis: clinical → treatment: doxycycline, amoxicillin, or cefuroxime → remember if lyme disease is left untreated, it can lead to musculoskeletal (joint), cardiovascular, or neurological disease.

- Watch for **morbiliform rashes** (hypersensitivity reaction) in patients using drugs such as PCN, sulfa, or phenytoin → rash is maculopapular in nature and **blanches with pressure** and appears similar to measles → treatment: diphenhydramine.

- Toxic epidermal necrolysis => a **drug-causing**, serious skin condition that presents with **nikolsky's sign** (skin peels off) → diagnosis: skin biopsy → treatment: manage in a designated burn center.

- Staphylococcal scaled skin syndrome => a **non-drug-causing** (rather, caused by *S. aureus*), serious skin condition that presents with **nikolsky's sign** (skin peels off) → diagnosis: skin biopsy → treatment: manage in a designated burn center + antibiotics (penicillin such as **nafcillin** or oxacillin).

- Toxic shock syndrome => caused *S. aureus* → involves the use of a **foreign material** (such as nasal packing cotton material in epistaxis) → *staph aureus* binds to the material and causes symptoms of shock (hypotension, fever, nausea, vomiting, altered mental status, renal failure, thrombocytopenia), desquamative rash, increased CPK, and LFTs → treatment: vigorous IVFs, vasopressors, and antibiotics (covering MRSA with vancomycin or linezolid).

- Pityriasis rosea => look for pruritus causing erythema and appear as a '**christmas tree**' or '**herald patch**' on the back → diagnosis: clinical; **negative VDRL** → treatment: self-limiting +/- diphenhydramine and topical steroids if symptoms persist longer than 2 months.

- Seborrheic dermatitis => due to *Pityrosporum ovale* causing excessive secretion of sebaceous content → presents with dandruff, and scaly skin, scalp, eyebrows, and scalp → treatment: **zinc pyrithione** as shampoo, topical steroids, topical ketoconazole, and selenium sulfide.

- Urticaria => pruritus < 24 hours → no hypotension or fever → treatment: antihistamine (diphenhydramine), cyproheptadine, or hydroxyzine → chronic treatment includes loratidine → some patients may require **desensitization** if interfering with normal activities → however, patients requiring desensitization while on **beta blocker** (propranolol) should have their beta blockers stopped before desensitization since beta blockers inhibit epinerphrine that may be much needed for an anaphylaxis reaction.

- Squamous cell carcinoma of the skin => look for ulceration of the lip → diagnosis: biopsy → treatment: surgical excision.

Chapter 4
Gastroenterology

Gastroesophageal Reflux Disease (GERD)

1. Etiology: Inappropriate relaxation of the lower esophageal sphincter.
2. Risk factors: The following conditions increase the risk of GERD: truncal obesity, pregnancy, hiatal hernia, alcohol, cigarette smoking, caffeine, chocolates, and spicy/fatty foods.
3. Findings: Upper epigatrium pain or burn sensation. Look for a patient who complains of epigastric pain that is triggered after meals and upon lying supine. Other symptoms are regurgitation, dysphagia, belching, nocturnal cough, sore throat, hoarseness, and asthma.
4. Diagnosis: Barium swallow initially, endoscopy with biopsy, and 24-hour ambulatory pH monitoring (**done in persistent or atypical cases).**
5. Treatment: Lifestyle changes => such as elevation of the head of the bed; do not eat trigger foods (coffee, alcohol, fatty foods, chocolate), and cigarettes. **Medications:** Start with antacids, H2 blockers, and 2-3 months of proton-pump inhibitors (PPIs) therapy.
6. **Refractory Cases:** Surgery (Nissen fundoplication or other type of repair).
7. Chronic GERD → leads to **Barret's Esophagus** (columnar metaplasia) → which leads to **esophageal adenocarcinoma** → perform endoscopy with biopsy to confirm Barret's Esophagus.
8. If Barret's Esophagus is suspected, enroll patient in **endoscopic surveillance program** for progression of dysplasia. If no dysplasia → perform EGD and biopsy every 2 years. If low-grade dysplasia → perform EGD and biopsy every 6 months to 1 year. If high-grade dysplasia → perform esophagectomy.

Peptic Ulcer Disease (PUD)

1. Peptic ulcer disease is mostly located in two sites: gastric and duodenum.
2. Causes: Major => Helicobacter Pylori (*H. Pylori*) and use of NSAIDS or aspirin. Minor => Zollinger-Ellison syndrome, HSV, and cytomegalovirus.
3. Findings: Patient usually complains of intermittent epigastric burning and abdominal pain. Other symptoms are nausea, vomiting, and upper GI bleed. May be relieved with **antacids or milk. Duodenal ulcers**: pain is relieved with/**after** food, and **gastric ulcers:** pain is worse with food.

4. Diagnosis: Endoscopy (biopsy and *H. Pylori* testing) with rapid urease testing for *H. Pylori*. To identify *H. Pylori* infection: Perform urease testing of sample, serum antibody, urea breath test (detects active infection), or fecal antigen test. Abdominal x-ray is used to assess complications such as perforation and gastric outlet obstruction.
5. Treatment: First, remember some medications may be contributing to PUD. Discontinue drugs such as NSAIDS or aspirin. Treat with H2 blockers or PPIs. For *H. Pylori* infection, use three or four-drug therapy as amoxicillin/ampicillin, clarithromycin, or metronidazole + proton-pump inhibitor (omeprazole) for 2 weeks. Bismuth may be added.
6. **Surgery:** indicated for refractory cases, perforations, upper GI bleed, gastric outlet obstruction, and Zollinger-Ellison syndrome.
7. Complication: **Perforation** (free air under diaphragm on abdominal film x-rays), **upper GI bleed**, and **gastric outlet obstruction**.
8. Atypical or non-healing ulcers may be due to Zollinger-Ellison syndrome (check gastrin levels) → treat with surgery.
9. Watch for signs of severe situation not PUD-related: age > 45, weight loss, anemia, and heme+ stool.

Achalasia

1. Etiology: Incomplete relaxation of lower esophageal sphincter (LES) and diminished peristalsis → Idiopathic; also, it may be due to *Chagas' disease* if from South America.
2. Findings: Dysphagia (solids + liquids). **No heartburn seen because no reflux or opening of LES**.
3. Diagnosis: Barium swallow shows **dilated esophagus + "bird-beak" narrowing**. Also **manometry** is used.
4. Treatment: Botulinum toxin injections, pneumatic balloon dilatation, calcium channel blockers, and surgery (myotomy-if no response).

Pancreatitis

1. Inflammation of the pancreas.
2. Etiologies: Most common causes are **gallstones** and **alcohol** (80% of cases). Others are: Trauma, hypertriglyceridemia, ERCP, viral (CMV, mumps, coxsackievirus), Hypercalcemia, and drugs (corticosteroids, thiazides, pentamidine, and sulfonamides).
3. Findings: **RUQ abdominal/midepigastric pain radiating to the back**, nausea, vomiting, and fever with leukocytosis. There may be Cullen's sign (periumbilical ecchymoses) and Grey Turner's sign (flank ecchymoses).

4. Diagnosis: Increased amylase and **lipase** (mostly), **increased ALT is seen in gallstone pancreatitis**, chest x-ray (to rule out pleural effusion), abdominal ultrasound (**if gallstone is suspected as cause**), and abdominal CT scan. Check 72-hour fecal fat (positive if greater than 7 g/day) in **chronic pancreatitis**.
5. Chronic pancreatitis: Due to idiopathic, alcohol, and cystic fibrosis. No involvement with gallstones.
6. Treatment: NPO, nasogastric tube (NGT), IVF, narcotics (**meperidine**) +/- antibiotics (imipenem or fluoroquinolone + metronidazole) for severe pancreatitis. **Do not use morphine** due to spasm of the sphincter of Oddi. **Treat chronic pancreatitis** with alcohol cessation, pancreatic enzyme replacement and fat-soluble vitamin supplements. **For gallstone pancreatitis**, treat with ERCP with papillotomy (if bile duct obstruction or cholangitis), then cholecystectomy when stable.
7. Complications: **Pseudocyst** (drain if symptomatic), pancreatic necrosis, pancreatic abscess, effusions, ARDS, and splenic vein thrombosis. Remember to consider malabsorption, diabetes, osteoporosis, and pancreatic cancer in complications with chronic pancreatitis.

Gallstone Disease

1. The most common cause of gallstone disease in U.S. is cholesterol stones.
2. Risk factors: "Female, forties, fertile, fat, and familial."
3. **Acalculous cholecystitis** occurs in the setting of trauma, burn, TPN **without gallstones**.
4. Findings: Gallstone disease is usually asymptomatic. Look for a 40something year old female who presents with nausea, vomiting, and right upper quadrant pain in the abdomen that causes radiation to her right shoulder after eating fatty foods. She may also complain of pain that wakes her up from sleep.
5. **Cholangitis:** a more serious condition than gallstones → infected bile → RUQ pain + fever + jaundice. Cholangitis includes Charcot's triad and Reynold's pentad. **Charcot's triad:** RUQ pain, jaundice, with fever and chills. **Reynolds' pentad:** Charcot's triad + altered mental status + shock.

Diagnosis:	Treatment:
You can start with labs: Look for increased (WBCs + amylase + LFTs), then use ultrasound, sensitive imaging for both gallstones and cholecystitis, and HIDA scan for an equivocal result on ultrasound.	Treat **acute cholecystitis** with NPO, IV antibiotics (cephalosporins), IVFs, and cholecystectomy within 72 hours/elective cholecystectomy/percutaneous biliary drain. For **cholangitis**: treat initially with admission, NPO, IVFs, and antibiotics (**ciprofloxacin**) → if the treatment is unsuccessful, you may use endoscopic sphincterotomy, ERCP with

	the use of stents, percutaneous transhepatic drainage, and surgical decompression. For **asymptomatic gallstones**: treat with elective/scheduled cholecystectomy.

Ulcerative Colitis

1. This is an inflammatory process. It presents as chronic and continuous (no skipped lesions) mucosal inflammation of the colon that extends proximally from the anus. Associated with **pyoderma gangrenosum**.
2. Findings: fatigue, abdominal pain, bloody diarrhea, weight loss, and anemia. Onset of flares may be triggered by cessation of smoking.
3. Diagnosis: CBC (anemia), BMP (electrolyte repletion), **p-ANCA**, negative stool cultures, barium enema (indicates lead-pipe colon with loss of haustra), and **colonoscopy with biopsy** (**confirms**; indicates ulceration with crypt abscess). Obtain abdominal x-ray to rule out complication of perforation or toxic megacolon.
4. Treatment: First with sulfasalazine; then steroids without or without azathioprine, 6-Mercaptopurine (6-MP), or methotrexate. In recurrent ulcerative colitis, use IV steroids, cyclosporine, or anti-TNF antibody. Surgery may be needed in cases of perforation or toxic megacolon.
5. Complication: **High-risk of colon cancer, toxic megacolon** (medical emergency; requires laparotomy), **perforation**.
6. Follow-up 8-10 years after diagnosis for surveillance colonoscopy with biopsy; then annually thereafter.

Crohn's Disease

1. Think of this as a bimodal distribution with peak occurring in the 20s age, and then between ages 50s and 70s. Involves any part of the GI tract, but mostly affects distal ileum & proximal colon → transmural inflammation pathology with **skipped lesions** pattern, linear ulcerations, and granulomas.
2. Findings: Fever, right lower quadrant (RLQ) abdominal pain, diarrhea (mostly without blood compared to ulcerative colitis, some mucus), anorexia, fatigue, weight loss, and anemia. **Associated with oral ulcers, anorectal fissures, perirectal abscess, fistulas**, and may **present similar to appendicitis** in children.
3. Diagnosis: CBC, ESR, LFT, iron, folate, vitamin B12, stool leukocytes, **positive ASCA**, colonoscopy with biopsy (confirms & shows **skipped lesions, noncaseating granuloma with mononuclear cell infiltrate**) , barium enema may be used (shows **cobblestoning, strictures, pseudodiverticula, fistulas, and**

abscess), CT scan may show abscess, and abdominal x-ray may show complication of perforation or toxic megacolon.

4. Treatment: First with sulfasalazine; then steroids, azathioprine, 6-mercaptopurine, or methotrexate. In recurrent cases, use IV steroids, cyclosporine, and anti-TNF antibody. **Surgery** may be needed in cases of perforation or toxic megacolon, and **stricturoplasty** to remove strictures.

5. Complication: **Intestinal obstruction**; **toxic megacolon or perforation** (medical emergency & requires laparatomy), intestinal fistulas to bowel, and abscesses. There is **lower risk** of colon cancer compared to ulcerative colitis.

6. Follow-up 8-10 years after diagnosis for surveillance colonoscopy with biopsy; then annually thereafter.

Hepatitis

1. Inflammation of the liver leading to acute or chronic liver diseases.
2. Etiologies: alcohol, viral, drug, ischemia, aspirin, pregnancy, and autoimmune.
3. Findings: **Acute** => nausea, vomiting, malaise, jaundice, RUQ pain and tenderness, hepatomegaly with **increased LFTs**; **chronic** => ascites, varices, palmar erythema, gynecomastia, spider angiomas, and testicular atrophy.
4. Diagnosis: Physical exam, increased LFTs, serology, PCR, abdominal ultrasound, and **liver biopsy** (confirms).
5. Treatment: Depends on the type of liver disease as indicated below. Along with the medical treatment, adopting some rest may help the acute symptoms.

Types of Liver Diseases:

- **Alcohol: increased LFTs** with AST > ALT (AST is more than twice as high as ALT). Treat with cessation of alcohol before it progresses to cirrhosis of the liver.

Viral:

- **Hepatitis A** => fecal-oral transmission with 6 days to 6 weeks incubation time duration → due to contaminated food, water → associated with daycare centers → diagnosis: IgM anti-HAV positive serology → treatment is supportive; patient may be asymptomatic.
- **Hepatitis B** => sexual, infected blood (needle), or perinatal transmission; and history of blood transfusion is another mode of transmission→ high-risk of transmission with IV drug users → 6 weeks to 6 months incubation time duration → **diagnosis**: increased LFTs and **serology**: IgM anti-HBc (first to appear, window phase), HBsAg-positive (acute/chronic), HBeAg (marker for infectivity); HBsAb means immunity from chronic infection or vaccination → **treatment**: **Lamivudine** +/- interferon. Complications: **cirrhosis** and **hepatocellular carcinoma with chronic infection**. **Prevention** is best achieved with

vaccination. Vaccinate patients with chronic hepatitis B against hepatitis A; use hepatitis B immunoglobulin for exposed neonates. Associated with **polyarteritis nodosa, glomerulonephritis**, and **arthritis**.

- **Hepatitis C => Most common** after **blood transfusion;** also IV drug use transmission → 6 weeks to 6 months incubation time duration → **diagnosis**: increased LFTs and serology: **HCV RNA**; HCV Ab only indicates **prior exposure** not recovery → **treatment: Ribavirin** +/- interferon → Complications: **cirrhosis** and **hepatocellular carcinoma with chronic infection**. Vaccinate patients with chronic hepatitis C against hepatitis A **and** hepatitis B. Associated with **cryoglobulinemia** and **membranoproliferative glomerulonephritis**.
- **Hepatitis D**: Coinfects patients with hepatitis B → transmission is same as hepatitis B → may lead to chronic infection → diagnosis: IgM Ab to hepatitis D antigen indicates recent resolution of infection and positive hepatitis D antigen indicates chronicity → treatment is similar to HBV. Risk of **fulminant hepatitis** and hepatocellular carcinoma.
- **Hepatitis E**: Transmission is similar to hepatitis A → diagnosis: Serology for HEV → treatment is supportive. Risk of **serious illness or fatality in pregnant women**.

Non-viral:

1. Drug-Induced hepatitis: **Acetaminophen toxicity** (acute within hours with nausea, vomiting, diaphoresis, pallor, RUQ pain, increased LFTs, and hepatomegaly) → treatment is supportive, activated charcoal, cholestyramine, and **acetylcysteine** (effective within 36 hours of ingestion). Other drugs that can cause drug-induced hepatitis: isoniazid, statins → treat by stopping offending drug.
2. Ischemic liver: Associated with underlying shock.
3. Aspirin-Induced (**Reye syndrome**): Occurs in children after the administration of Aspirin for fever.
4. Pregnancy-related (Acute fatty liver of pregnancy): Onset is usually in the 3rd trimester → treat with **emergency delivery**.
5. Autoimmune Hepatitis: Idiopathic; seen in middle-aged women → **positive anti-smooth muscle antibodies** or **antinuclear antibodies (ANA)** → treatment: corticosteroids.

Cirrhosis + Ascites

1. This is a chronic process involving fibrotic and irreversible changes of the liver that may lead to hepatocellular carcinoma.
2. Etiologies: Alcohol (happens to be the most common cause of cirrhosis in U.S), viral hepatitis, hemochromatosis, Wilson's disease, and alpha1 antitrypsin deficiency.

3. Findings: Look for these: Ascites, varices, palmar erythema, gynecomastia, spider angiomas, and testicular atrophy. Symptoms indicating abnormal liver function may include edema, jaundice, and coagulopathy. Fibrosis of the liver leads to portal hypertension (**esophageal varices & splenomegaly**), and **encephalopathy** indicates diminished liver function and portal hypertension. Others may be initially asymptomatic.

4. Diagnosis: AST, ALT, CBC, PT/PTT, platelets, abdominal ultrasound/CT scan (to assess cirrhosis, nodules, & ascites), **liver biopsy** (to evaluate liver damage), and **paracentesis** for ascites (diagnostic & therapeutic; to evaluate cell count, differential, bacterial cultures, acid-fast stain, cytology, & albumin). For **serum-ascites albumin gradient, SAAG greater than/equal to 1.1** includes cirrhosis, heart failure, and hepatic vein thrombosis. **SAAG less than/equal to 1.1** includes pancreatitis, cancer, nephrotic syndrome, peritonitis, and trauma.

5. Coagulopathy may show increased PT & PTT. Treat coagulopathy with fresh frozen plasma (FFP). **Vitamin K** should not be used; because it is ineffective with a damaged liver.

6. Treatment: Advise cessation of alcohol consumption; Ascites may be treated with diuretics (furosemide) & spironolactone. TIPS (shunt) have been used for ascites, but may precipitate encephalopathy. Hepatic encephalopathy is associated with hyperammonemia; so treat with **lactulose** and **neomycin**. Low protein diet may be required for refractory encephalopathy. **Liver transplantation** is usually indicated for certain candidates-depending of severity of liver damage.

7. Complications: **Spontaneous bacterial peritonitis (SBP)** associated with worsening fever, abdominal pain, ascites, altered mental status, and hepatic encephalopathy. Diagnose with positive bacterial cultures (due to *Escherichia Coli or Strep Pneumoniae*) or peritoneal fluid with **neutrophil count > 250**. Treat first with **third-generation cephalosporin (cefotaxime)** or fluoroquinolone. Other complications are hepatorenal syndrome (kidney failure as a result of liver failure) and DIC.

Upper GI Bleed

1. To locate the site of bleeding, the ligament of Treitz is a great reference point. Bleeding of the upper GI which is located proximal to the reference point, ligament of Treitz.

2. Etiologies: Peptic ulcer disease, varices, gastritis, and Mallory-Weiss tears.

3. Findings: Nausea, vomiting of blood (hematemesis), dizziness, lightheadedness, abdominal pain, and passing dark, tarry stools (**melena**). May also present with signs of shock: pallor, hypotension, and tachycardia.

4. Diagnosis: Stabilize the patient by assessing the ABCs; check vitals, hematocrit (may be normal initially), **BUN/creatinine** (an **elevated BUN** with normal creatinine = **GI blood loss**). Place **NG tube and lavage**, **endoscopy** (diagnostic & therapeutic).

5. Treatment: Stabilize the patient by assessing the ABCs. Use two large-bore needles for IV access and replace blood products. Treat variceal bleeds initially with **octreotide, sclerotherapy,** or **band ligation**; if severe, use **balloon tamponade, embolization,** or TIPS. For variceal prophylaxis, use **propranolol** (non-selective beta blocker). Surgery (consult) may be needed for refractory or persistent bleeding.
6. Bleeding due to peptic ulcer disease may be treated with endoscopic epinephrine injection and PPIs. Eradicate for *H. Pylori*.
7. Mallory-Weiss tears: Bleeding may stop it spontaneously.
8. Avoid offending agents causing bleeding in gastritis such as NSAIDs, aspirin. Treat with H2 antagonists and PPIs.

Lower GI Bleed

1. Bleeding of the lower GI which is located distal to the reference point, ligament of Treitz.
2. Etiologies: **Diverticulosis** (**most common cause**), vascular ectasia, colon cancer, inflammatory bowel disease, enteritis, colitis, and hemorrhoids.
3. Findings: Bright red blood per rectum (hematochezia), tenesmus, diarrhea.
4. Diagnosis: Rectal exam (for hemorrhoids or fissures). Rule out upper GI bleed with NGT and lavage, **endoscopy**; then **colonoscopy** (therapeutic), **radionuclide RBC scans** (for slow bleeds and usually if colonoscopy did not help), and **angiography/arteriography/exploratory laparotomy** (for rapid bleeds or **refractory cases**; used for embolization therapy).
5. Treatment: Stabilize the patient. Check vital signs and hemoglobin level. Give IVFs and blood. Diagnose; monitor vitals and hemoglobin level every 4-8 hours. **Remember:** bleeding may stop spontaneously in diverticulosis. If not, epinephrine injection, vasopressin, or embolization. **Surgery** (resection of affected bowel).
6. **THINK: Blood in stool/rectum =>** Colon cancer (**"occult"** blood), diverticulosis (**painless** lower GI bleed), and hemorrhoids (**"streaks"** of blood). **A positive occult blood or lower GI bleed in a patient > 40 years old is colon cancer until proven otherwise.**
7. **Complications** for diverticulosis are hemorrhage and diverticulitis (LLQ pain, fever, increased WBCs, and diarrhea/constipation). Treat diverticulitis with IVF, NPO, and antibiotics.

GASTROENTEROLOGY 1-LINER JUNKY CASES

- Odynophagia => pain with swallowing → if thrush, think HIV, HSV, CMV (with CD4 < 50) → treat first with fluconazole; if there are ulcers (HSV), treat with acyclovir. Endoscopy with biopsy may be used if there's no improvement.
- Pill esophagitis => inflammation of esophagus due to drugs (doxycycline, quinidine, alendronate, NSAIDs) → diagnose with **air contrast barium swallow** → treat by stopping offending agent.
- **Mallory-Weiss tears** => superficial esophageal tears that may bleed → symptoms: vomiting & retching in an alcoholic or bulimic patient → diagnosis: endoscopy with biopsy → treat with sclerotherapy or band ligation.
- **Boorhave tears** => esophageal ruptures caused by vomiting & retching in an alcoholic or bulimic patient → may be iatrogenic from endoscopic procedure → diagnosis: **water-soluble contrast**, endoscopy → treat with **surgical repair**.
- Long-standing heartburn or reflux is the cause of **peptic stricture.**
- **Plummer-Vinson syndrome** => esophageal web + iron deficiency anemia → may be associated with esophageal cancer.
- Scleroderma → autoimmune, positive ANA → Findings: mask-like face + heartburn + Raynaud's phenomenon (**CREST** syndrome: **C**alcinosis cutis, **R**aynaud's phenomenon, **E**sophageal dysmotility, **S**clerodactyly, and **T**elangiectasias) → due to fibrosis and atrophy of smooth muscle.
- **Zenker's diverticulum** => outpouching of the esophagus → Findings: dysphagia + regurgitation + foul smelling (halitosis) breath → diagnosis: barium swallow.
- **Diffuse esophageal spasm or nutcracker esophagus** => atypical chest pains due to esophageal contractions → diagnosis: manometry → treat with calcium channel blockers and surgery (myotomy).
- **Aorto-enteric fistula** => causes "**massive**" lower GI bleed after aortic graft placement → treatment: laparotomy.
- Primary biliary cirrhosis => autoimmune, middle-aged woman → destruction of intrahepatic bile ducts → Findings: pruritus, jaundice, malabsorption, osteoporosis → diagnosis: **positive antimitochondrial antibodies (AMA)**, increased alkaline phosphatase, increased bilirubin, and biopsy (confirms) → treat with **ursodeoxycholic acid, cholestyramine** (for symptomatic pruritus), fat-soluble vitamins, and liver transplantation (last resort).
- Primary sclerosing cholangitis => Occurs in young-adult patients with ulcerative colitis → intrahepatic + extrahepatic fibrosis of bile ducts → Findings: RUQ pain + pruritus or asymptomatic; may present like cholangitis → diagnosis: increased alkaline phosphatase, increased bilirubin, positive AMSA and p-ANCA, and ERCP shows beaded strictures → treat with **ursodeoxycholic acid, cholestyramine** (for symptomatic pruritus), fat-soluble vitamins, stenting of the beaded strictures, and liver transplantation (last resort).
- **Cholangitis** => infected bile → RUQ pain + fever + jaundice → diagnosis: ERCP

(& therapeutic with endoscopic sphincterotomy) → treat initially with admission, NPO, IVFs, and antibiotics (**ciprofloxacin**) → if no response, treat with endoscopic sphincterotomy/stent placement, percutaneous transhepatic drainage, or decompression.

- **Autoimmune hepatitis** => autoimmune; affects young women → diagnosis: increased LFTs, ANA, **anti-smooth muscle** antibody (ASMA), liver biopsy (confirms) → treat with steroids + azathioprine.
- Wilson's disease => autosomal recessive; **copper overload** → Findings: neurological symptoms + **Kayser-Fleischer rings** (due to deposits in **basal ganglia**) → diagnosis: increased urinary copper, low serum ceruloplasmin, and liver biopsy shows copper → treat with chelation (penicillamine, trientine).
- Hereditary hemochromatosis => autosomal recessive; **iron overload**-deposits in organs causing cirrhosis/liver cancer, diabetes, dilated cardiomyopathy → Findings: hyperpigmented/bronze skin, increased LFTs, arthritis, diabetes, heart failure → diagnosis: **increased** (iron saturation, ferritin, and transferrin saturation) and HFE gene mutation → treat with **phlebotomy** + genetic counseling.
- Alpha1-antitrypsin disorder → autosomal recessive; causes cirrhosis of the liver + emphysema of the lung → diagnosis: chest x-ray, low or absent of alpha1-antitrypsin on serum protein electrophoresis (SPEP), genotype analysis → treat by replacing alpha1-antitrypsin + liver transplantation.
- **Irritable bowel syndrome (IBS)** => autonomic disorder; associated with psychosocial stressors; **diagnosis of exclusion** → Findings: abdominal pain + bloating + altered bowel function with diarrhea/constipation + feeling of incomplete relief of defecation → diagnosis: Labs (CBC, BMP, TSH, stool ova & parasites) → treat with high fiber diet, increased water intake, antidepressants (TCAs) may help, and dicyclomine/hyoscamine for postprandial symptoms such as abdominal cramps.
- **Diarrhea** => depending on the cause and timing of the onset (acute = < 2 weeks, chronic = > 4 weeks) → **osmotic** (lactose intolerance, mannitol), **secretory** (toxins: e.g. cholera, VIPoma), **infectious** (*E. coli, Shigella, Salmonella, Campylobacter, Clostridium difficile* bacteria), **exudative** (mucosal inflammation due to IBD), **systemic** (hyperthyroidism, viral illness), and **malabsorption** (celiac sprue with dermatitis herpetiformis) → diagnosis: if there's fever, check **fecal leukocytes, bacterial leukocytes**; rectal exam; check for occult blood in stool; stool for bacteria, ova, and parasites; WBCs; fat levels; and *Clostridium difficile* toxin; **osmotic gap** may be calculated with **290 − 2 (stool Na + stool K)** → treatment is with oral and IV fluids, electrolyte repletion, **loperamide** for diarrhea, and **dicyclomine/hyoscamine** for postprandial symptoms (abdominal cramps) → treat *C. difficile* with metronidazole, vancomycin.
- *Gardial lambia* infection => fatty, greasy, malodorous → protozoal cysts → treat with metronidazole.
- Other causes of diarrhea are: factitious diarrhea from laxative use by a medical staff, diabetes (diabetic diarrhea), and hyperthyroidism (systemic).
- Celiac sprue => autoimmune, familial → due to wheat, rye → associated with iron deficiency anemia, osteoporosis (due to vitamin D deficiency) → Findings: chronic diarrhea + malabsorption + weight loss → diagnosis: **histology of small**

bowel (flattening or loss of villi + inflammation), **antibody assay** (antiendomysial antibody/anti-tissue transglutaminase) → treat with **gluten-free diet** (found in grains).

Chapter 5
Hematology
Anemia

1. Defined as the decrease in hemoglobin of less than 12 mg/dL in women and less than 14 mg/dL in men.
2. Etiologies: Focus on the main causes. They are: **Blood loss** (trauma, surgery, GI bleed, heavy menstrual cycles), **medications** (phenytoin, methyldopa, chloramphenicol, and sulfa drugs), **alcoholism, hereditary** (hemophilia, G6PD), and **anemia due to chronic diseases** (cancer, chronic inflammation and rheumatological diseases).
3. Findings: Pallor, fatigue, dizziness, light-headedness, palpitations, tachycardia, chest pains, systolic ejection murmurs and syncope. Watch for positive stool guaiac in lower GI bleed; and pancytopenia in malignancy, toxins, radiation, and myelodysplasia.
4. Diagnosis: Start with: CBC with differential, mean corpuscular volume (MCV), reticulocyte index or count (> 2% = anemia), and peripheral blood smear. Then, secondary tests include iron studies (ferritin, TIBC, serum iron), serum folate, serum B12, TSH, hemolysis labs (**increased** unconjugated bilirubin, **low** haptoglobin, **increased** LDH, Coomb's test), and DIC hemolysis panel.
5. Treatment: For emergency: identify bleeding source, IVFs + blood transfusions with packed RBCs. Others: ferrous sulfate, erythropoietin, folate, and vitamin B12. Treat the underlying cause of anemia. Maintain hemoglobin > 8 mg/dL.
6. Anemia can be classified into **microcytic** (MCV less than 80), **normocytic** (MCV between 80-100), **or macrocytic** (MCV greater than 80).

Microcytic Anemia

1. Look for MCV less than 80 fL.
2. Etiologies: Iron deficiency anemia, Lead poisoning, Anemia of chronic disease, Sideroblastic anemia, and Thalassemia. **THINK: I - L. A. S. T.**
3. **Iron deficiency anemia:** Most common cause of anemia in U.S. → **symptoms** may include **pallor, pica**, melena, bright red blood per rectum, positive fecal occult blood (guaiac positive), irregular or heavy menstrual cycles, and **family history of thalassemia** → **diagnose** with CBC, iron studies (**low iron, low ferritin, increased total iron-binding capacity, TIBC;** also note: **low TIBC saturation**), and peripheral blood smear; **wide/increased RDW** → **treat** by identifying the underlying cause; give oral iron supplementation, parenteral iron

therapy for GI diseases, and erythropoietin (Epogen) for anemia of chronic disease.

4. **Lead poisoning:** Affects children living in old or abandoned building → **symptoms** include vomiting, **ataxia, colicky abdominal pain, seizures, irritability,** and **encephalopathy with cerebral edema** → **diagnose** with serum lead levels, increased free erythrocyte protoporphyrin, and **peripheral blood smear** shows **basophilic RBC stippling.**

5. **Anemia of chronic disease:** Identify underlying chronic illness (malignancy, inflammation) → **diagnose** with low iron, low TIBC, **increased ferritin** (due to increased acute-phase reactants) → **treat** underlying cause and erythropoietin.

6. **Sideroblastic anemia:** Etiologies are drugs (chloramphenicol, isoniazid, chronic alcohol use, and lead poisoning) → **diagnose** with low iron, **increased** ferritin, and **normal** TIBC, peripheral blood smear shows **normal and dimorphic RBCs with basophilic stippling,** bone marrow biopsy confirms with **erythroid hyperplasia and ringed sideroblasts,** and **Prussian blue stain** (most accurate) → **treat** with **pyridoxine** and stop the offending drug or agent.

7. **Thalassemia:** Decreased synthesis of alpha-globin or beta-globin protein subunits; when 4 alleles of alpha subunit are affected, there's risk of **hydrops fetalis** → **symptoms** include splenomegaly and anemia in alpha thalassemia; **bone deformities, growth retardation,** jaundice, and hepatosplenomegaly in beta thalassemia → diagnose with family history, peripheral blood smear shows **target cells,** nucleated RBCs, or diffuse basophilia, x-ray of skull showing "crew-cut" or "hair-on-end" appearance, **electrophoresis** confirms with **increased hemoglobin A2** or **hemoglobin F** → no treatment needed for asymptomatic minor thalassemia; treat major thalassemia with **blood transfusions** and iron chelation therapy (**deferoxamine**) to prevent hemochromatosis or secondary hemosiderosis. No iron supplementation due to risk of iron overload.

Normocytic Anemia

1. Look for MCV between 80-100 fL.
2. Etiologies: Acute blood loss, hemolytic anemia (microangiopathic hemolytic anemia, autoimmune hemolytic anemia, sickle cell disease, G6PD deficiency, hereditary spherocytosis, paroxysmal nocturnal hemoglobinuria), anemia of chronic disease, end-stage renal disease, and aplastic anemia.
3. **Acute blood loss:** Usually as a result of trauma (hemorrhage) → symptoms include hypotension, cold and pale skin, and tachycardia → diagnosis is usually clinical; identify source of bleeding → treat with blood transfusion. Hemoglobin may be normal initially, so transfuse anyway.
4. **Hemolytic anemia:** Diagnose with **increased** reticulocyte count, **increased** unconjugated bilirubin, **increased** LDH, **low** haptoglobin. Examples are below:
5. **Microangiopathic hemolytic anemia:** Intravascular hemolysis → presents in DIC, HUS, TTP → diagnose with schistocytes, helmet cells, and fragmented

RBCs on peripheral blood smear → treat underlying condition. See below.

6. **Autoimmune hemolytic anemia:** Seen in leukemia/lymphoma (mycoplasma, CLL), drugs (methyldopa, penicillin), lupus or lupus-causing drugs → diagnose with spherocytes (incomplete macrophage destruction) on peripheral blood smear and **positive Coomb's test** → treat with steroids, IVIG, and splenectomy.

7. **Sickle cell anemia:** Autosomal recessive disease, family history → symptoms include fever, bone pains, palpitations, pallor, dyspnea, splenomegaly → diagnosis: peripheral blood smear shows **sickled cells**, howell-jolly bodies, and hemolysis; **hemoglobin electrophoresis** (definitive diagnostic test) → treat with oxygen, IVFs, anagelsics, antibiotics, blood transfusions, folic acid supplementation, **hydroxyurea (for recurrent crises)**, **exchange transfusion (for acute chest syndrome/pulmonary infarcts, retinal infarcts, priapism)**, and bone marrow transplantation. Avoid precipitating factors such as hypoxia, dehydration, stress, and high altitude. **Complications** include acute chest crisis, **pulmonary infarcts**, **sickle cell cardiomyopathy**, papillary necrosis, acute renal failure, spontaneous abortions, **avascular necrosis**, infections, and aplastic crisis. Vaccinate all patients from encapsulated bacterials (*Haemophilus influenza*, *Streptococcus pneumonia*, and hepatitis B virus).

8. **G6PD deficiency:** X-linked recessive trait → sudden hemolysis after exposure to **fava beans**, **drugs** (sulfa, antimalarials, salicylates), infection → diagnosis: peripheral blood smear shows bite cells and Heinz bodies and **RBC enzyme assay** (note: G6PD may be normal initially, but decreases later) → treat by discontinuing and avoiding triggering foods and drugs.

9. **Hereditary spherocytosis:** Family history, autosomal dominant → diagnose with **spherocytes** on peripheral blood smear, splenomegaly, increased mean corpuscular hemoglobin concentration (MCHC), and **positive osmotic fragility test** (confirms) → treat with splenectomy.

10. **Paroxysmal nocturnal hemoglobinuria (PNH):** Associated with pancytopenia, recurrent thrombosis → diagnosis: flow cytometry, **CD 55 and CD 59** (most accurate; decay accelerating factor), **sugar-water** and **Ham's test** → treatment: steroids → risk of AML and aplastic anemia.

11. **End-stage renal disease:** Renal failure causing anemia → treat with erythropoietin (Epogen).

12. **Aplastic anemia:** Consider the following malignancy, radiation, benzene, chemotherapy, medications (carbamezapine, chloramphenicol, zidovudine) → diagnosis: decreased reticulocytes, WBCs, and platelets → treat by stopping offending drugs, antithymocyte globulin (ATG), or bone marrow transplantation.

Macrocytic Anemia

1. Look for MCV greater than 100 fL.
2. Etiologies: Folate deficiency, vitamin B12 deficiency.
3. **Folate deficiency:** Caused by poor dietary intake (from tea & toast diet), chronic

alcoholism, drugs (phenytoin, methotrexate, TMP-SMX, zidovudine, some chemotherapy medications), hypothyroidism, and malabsorption → diagnosis: serum/RBC folate level, peripheral blood smear shows **oval macrocytes and hypersegmented neutrophils** → treat by reducing alcohol consumption, discontinuing drugs, and give **oral folate**.

4. **Vitamin B12 deficiency:** Due to **pernicious anemia** (anti-parietal cell antibodies), gastrectomy, strict vegetarian diet, terminal ileum resection or dysfunction, chronic pancreatitis, and *Diphyllobothrium latum* infection → symptoms include **neurologic deficits** (**loss of sensation, ataxia gait, dementia, hyperreflexia**, paresthesias, and positive Babinski) → diagnosis: serum levels of vitamin B12, **intrinsic factor antibody** and **anti-parietal cell antibody** for pernicious anemia, **schilling test**; increased homocysteine levels; use **methylmalonic acid levels** to confirm diagnosis in patients with borderline results of B12 levels → treat with **monthly** vitamin B12 injections.

Disseminated Intravascular Coagulation (DIC)

1. Medical emergency with an underlying condition causing the activation of coagulation system.
2. Etiologies: **pregnancy** or **obstetric** complications, malignancy, sepsis, shock, or trauma.
3. Findings: Bleeding from puncture or IV sites, **thrombosis (risk)**.
4. Diagnosis: **Increased** prothrombin time (PT), partial thromboplastin (PTT), and bleeding time (BT); increased fibrin degradation products, decreased fibrin, decreased clotting factors, thrombocytopenia, positive D-dimer test, and hemolysis with schistocytes on peripheral blood smear.
5. Treatment: Treat the underlying condition, **FFP**, or **cryoprecipitate** (for fibrinogen replacement). Avoid platelet transfusions only with severe bleeding. **Heparin** may be needed in rare cases for thrombosis. Give antibiotics when necessary.

Hemolytic Uremic Syndrome (HUS)

1. Usually found in children due to *E. Coli* **O157:H7** infection or viral illness.
2. Triad => **H**emolytic anemia + **A**cute renal failure + **T**hrombocytopenia → **THINK: H.A.T.**
3. Findings: Abdominal pain, diarrhea in children after eating "hamburger at a

picnic."
4. Diagnosis: Usually clinical; but peripheral blood smear shows hemolysis with schistocytes and helmet cells.
5. Treatment: Supportively +/- dialysis and/or transfusions.

Thrombotic Thrombocytopenic Purpura (TTP)

1. Etiologies: Some of the causes of TTP are: Pregnancy, HIV, and drugs such as ticlopidine and OCPs.
2. Findings: **THINK: H. A. T + Fever/Neuro => Pentad: H**emolytic anemia + **A**cute renal failure + **T**hrombocytopenia + fever + neurological problems (headaches, confusion).
3. Diagnosis: Consider a peripheral blood smear: shows hemolysis with schistocytes and helmet cells.
4. Treatment: **Plasmapheresis** or **FFP**. No platelets as they may worsen TTP.

Polycythemia Vera (PCV)

1. Myeloproliferative syndrome causing **increased RBCs.**
2. **Chronic hypoxia** is the most known cause of erythrocytosis secondary to lung disease (differentiates from primary PCV).
3. Findings: watch for a man (usually) who has **pruritus** after taking a hot bath/shower with malaise, fever, **plethora, splenomegaly**, headaches, blurred vision, large retinal veins, stroke, MI, and hepatic vein thrombosis.
4. Diagnosis: **increased hematocrit** and **RBC mass > 50%, low** erythropoietin level (increased in chronic hypoxia-induced polycythemia), ABG, increased LAP and B12 levels. **Bone marrow biopsy** confirms diagnosis with **hypercellular** marrow. Other test: **positive JAK-2**.
5. Treatment: **Series of phlebotomy + aspirin; hydroxyurea**; and anagrelide (reduces platelets & risk of thrombosis).
6. **Complications:** Risk of conversion to acute myelogenous leukemia (AML) or other myeloproliferative syndrome.

Hypercoagulable State

1. Predisposes patients to clotting and thrombotic events.

2. Inherited: **Factor V Leiden deficiency (most common,** associated with homocysteine), homocysteinemia, protein C, protein S, prothrombin 20210 gene mutation, and anti-thrombin III deficiency.

3. Acquired: Look for association with risk factors of deep venous thrombosis (DVT): immobilization, obesity, smoking, pregnancy, malignancy, DIC, birth control pills (OCPs); nephrotic syndrome; lupus anticoagulant (antiphospholipid antibody syndrome), homocysteine, and inflammatory bowel disease (due to low protein S and cytokines).

4. **Test the following groups for hypercoagulable test:** Presence of DVT in a patient < 50 years old, first-degree relative with thrombotic events before 50 years old, recurrent episodes of venous thromboses, and in patient with increased homocysteine levels.

5. **Diagnosis:** Screening include activated protein C (APC) resistance (for factor V Leiden deficiency), antithrombin deficiency, protein C deficiency, protein S deficiency, prothrombin gene mutation, antiphospholipid antibody, and homocysteine levels. Also diagnose DVT with **venous duplex ultrasound of the lower extremities** or MRI. D-dimer assay can be used for patients with low pretest probability for DVT.

6. **Treatment:** Heparin, low-molecular-weight heparin, warfarin, inferior vena cava (IVC) filter. First time thromboses are treated for 3-6 months. Lifetime therapy of warfarin is indicated for antiphospholipid syndrome, antithrombin deficiency, > 2 spontaneous thromboses. Watch for heparin-induced and warfarin-induced skin necroses. Warfarin-induced skin necrosis is due to **protein C deficiency**. Bridge warfarin with heparin for 3-5 days until INR reaches typically, targeted therapeutic goal of 2-3.

7. **Pregnant patients** with previous thrombotic episodes may be treated with low-molecular-weight heparin.

8. Complications of DVT => pulmonary embolism, post-obstructive syndrome (pain + edema only in affected leg), and chronic venous insufficiency.

9. Absolute contraindications for anticoagulation: Active bleeding, platelets < 20,000, and in intracranial bleeding or neurosurgical procedure in the last 10 days.

Platelet Disorders

1. Usually involves disorders with thrombocytopenia (decreased platelets) or platelet dysfunction that predisposes patients to bleeding.

2. Findings: **Petechiae**, ecchymosis, easy bruising, **epistaxis**, and bleeding involving the gingival and GI tract.

3. Diagnosis: Depends on the platelet disorders; may include CBC, peripheral blood smear, platelet count post-transfusion, and bone marrow biopsy may show thrombocytopenia.

4. **Platelet disorders include**: Heparin-induced, idiopathic thrombocytopenic purpura, drug-induced, HUS, and TTP.

5. **Heparin-induced thrombocytopenia (HIT):** Immune-mediated → occurs usually around day 5 after use; may occur with presence of **skin necrosis** (IV site) → diagnosis: **platelet factor-4 (PF-4) antibodies** → treat by stopping heparin immediately and starting direct thrombin inhibitors (lepirudin or argatroban) → if HIT occurs with IV unfractionated heparin instead, just stop the drug!

6. **Idiopathic thrombocytopenic purpura (ITP):** Associated with IgG antibodies → may occur prior to an upper respiratory infection → diagnosis: low platelets & may have increased bleeding time; ultrasound (to check spleen); antibodies to glycoprotein 2b/3a receptor; bone marrow biopsy (increased megakaryocytes); may also be diagnosis of exclusion → treat with **steroids, IVIG,** and **splenectomy** (last resort if unresponsive).

7. **Drug-induced thrombocytopenia:** Due to drugs (sulfa drugs, quinine, antibiotics, glycoprotein IIb/IIIa inhibitors, **linezolid**, clopidogrel) → diagnosis is clinical and by stopping the offending drug → treatment is by avoiding offending drug.

8. **Platelet dysfunction:** Usually normal platelet count → may be **acquired or inherited. Acquired:** includes liver disease, DIC, **chronic renal disease**, chronic use of aspirin, and multiple myeloma → if bleeding occurs, treat with **desmopressin, FFP/cryoprecipitate,** and OCPs (for women with heavy menstrual cycles). **Inherited:** includes Bernard-Soulier syndrome and Glanzmann's thrombasthenia → if bleeding occurs, treat with **desmopressin** and **FFP/cryoprecipitate.**

9. **ITP + autoimmune hemolytic anemia** (with spherocytes and positive Coomb's test) => **Evans syndrome**.

10. **Platelet transfusion:** Transfuse platelets when < 15,000 even if asymptomatic and when < 50,000 with symptoms or there is an ongoing bleeding. Any asymptomatic patient with a minimum of 50,000 platelet count **does not** need platelet transfusion.

***Always rule out pseudothrombocytopenia by rechecking platelets in citrated blood.**

Coagulopathies

1. Coagulopathies involve abnormal clotting cascades with risk of hemorrhaging.
2. Etiologies: Drugs (warfarin, heparin, and enoxaparin), vitamin K deficiency (secondary to alcoholism, antibiotic use, malnutrition).
3. Findings: Deep bleeding (hemarthrosis) into joints, muscles, GI tract, and GU tract.
4. Diagnosis: History of drugs, perform physical exam for liver disease, order PT/PTT. If increased PTT = abnormality in intrinsic pathway (factors VIII, IX, XI, XII). If increased PT = abnormality in extrinsic pathway (factor VII). If both PT and PTT increased = abnormality in combined pathway (factors V, X, II).

5. Treatment: Stop precipitating drugs (heparin, warfarin, etc). **FFP** (for bleeding). Replace vitamin K when needed.

Von Willerbrand's Disease (vWD)

1. A bleeding disorder that is inherited as autosomal-dominant. Check family history.
2. Findings: Mucocutaneous bleeding, joint bleeding, **increased bleeding time (BT)**.
3. Diagnosis: **Low levels of vWF antigen**, increased PTT, and **abnormal ristocetin cofactor activity** (vWF activity).
4. Treatment: **Desmopressin** => used to stop bleeding + prevent bleeding in surgical procedure.

Hemophilia A & B

1. A bleeding disorder that is inherited as X-linked recessive → history of bleeding in family members or noted carriers in family members.
2. Findings: Deep bleeding (hemarthrosis) into joints, muscles, GI tract, and GU tract.
3. Diagnosis: **Increased** partial thromboplastin time (**PTT**). If PTT is increased, proceed with **mixing study** with normal plasma. If corrected, then suggests factor deficiency. Then obtain **quantitative Factor VIII/IX levels** and **activity**. If lab results confirm hemophilia A, but no family history, may need to obtain vWD level.
4. Treatment: Factor VIII (in hemophilia A), factor IX (in hemophilia B).

Blood Transfusion Complications

1. Delayed hemolysis: Occurs several days (4-14) after transfusion → symptoms include fever, jaundice, anemia, and hemoglobinuria → diagnosis: low hemoglobin, increased LDH, increased unconjugated bilirubin, and microspherocytes on peripheral blood smear → treat with acetaminophen for fever and type and screen blood for future transfusions.
2. ABO incompatibility → occurs during blood transfusion → symptoms include hemolytic anemia + hypotension + tachycardia.
3. Anaphylaxis: due to **response to plasma proteins** (for example: fresh frozen plasma) → symptoms include hypotension, **urticaria, wheezing**, flushing, chest

pains, edema, and shock **without hemolysis** → diagnosis: clinical → treat with IV epinephrine and **saline-washed packed RBCs** for future transfusions → seen in patients with **IgA deficiency**.

4. Transfusion-related acute lung injury → look for a patient with shortness of breath few minutes after a blood transfusion + chest x-ray with infiltrates.

HEMATOLOGY 1-LINER JUNKY CASES

- Cold agglutinin disease => associated with mycoplasma infection + mononucleosis → acrocyanosis in cold exposure → positive cold agglutinin test.
- Mechanical heart valves => produce hemolyzed RBCs.
- Eosinophilia => think atopy, allergy, eczema, parasitic infection, and pulmonary eosinophilia (Loffler syndrome).
- Basophilia => **proliferative myelopoiesis** and allergies.
- HELLP => **H**emolysis + **E**levated **L**iver enzymes + **L**ow **P**latelets in microangiopathic hemolytic anemia.
- Cryoprecipitate => **contains fibrinogen + factor 8**.
- Do **not** transfuse an **asymptomatic** patient with blood! Transfuse only if symptomatic.
- Give **washed RBCs** to IgA deficiency patients. The RBCs are washed and free of traces of plasma, WBCs, and platelets.
- Whole blood => usually given in emergency for massive, acute blood loss.
- **Increased bleeding time => platelet dysfunction**.
- **Increased thrombin time => defect in the cross-linking of fibrin** (e.g. DIC).
- Essential thrombocytosis => essentially increased platelets (> 600K) with other normal labs.
- Scurvy (vitamin C deficiency) => **normal labs** (platelets, BT, PT, PTT, and RBC count) + petechiae + bleeding gums + fingernail and gum hemorrhages → treat with oral vitamin C.
- Measurement of ferritin can differentiate iron deficiency anemia (low ferritin) from thalassemia (normal ferritin).
- Desmopressin => used to stop bleeding + preventing bleeding in surgical procedure.

Chapter 6
Oncology
Acute Lymphocytic Leukemia (ALL)

1. A type of leukemia that affects mostly children → ALL → associated with Down syndrome.
2. Findings: Petechiae, purpura, pallor, pancytopenia (anemia, neutropenia, thrombocytopenia), flu-like symptoms (fever, malaise, URI, sorethroat, lethargy), bone pain with limping/inability to walk, and bleeding with easy bruising. Other signs of extramedullary spread are **lymphadenopathy, enlarged spleen and liver, and testicular/CNS symptoms**.
3. Diagnosis: **Labs:** Usually **increased WBCs** (may be decreased), **decreased platelets, increased uric acid**, and **increased LDH → peripheral blood smear: increased lymphocytes → bone marr-ow biopsy** (confirms), (CALLA+, TdT+, determines prognosis) → **Chest x-ray, CT scan** (mediastinal processes and brain metastases), **and lumbar puncture**.
4. Treatment: Combination chemotherapy: **Vincristine + prednisone + daunorubicin** to induce remission → **methotrexate or 6-mercaptopurine** to maintain remission. Prognosis is based on age of onset + cytogenic studies. Many children achieve complete remission.

Acute Myelogenous Leukemia (AML)

1. A type of leukemia that affects mostly adults.
2. Related to **smoking, radiation, chemotherapy drugs,** and **benzene**.
3. Findings: Same as ALL → Petechiae, purpura, pallor, pancytopenia (anemia, neutropenia, thrombocytopenia), lethargy, fever, and bleeding with easy bruising. Other symptoms: **disseminated intravascular coagulation (DIC) and gingival hyperplasia**.
4. Diagnosis: **decreased LAP, increased** myelocytic cells, **increased** uric acid. **Peripheral blood smear:** myeloblasts, **Auer rods. Bone marrow biopsy** (confirms blasts by positive **myeloperoxidase staining**).
5. Treatment: **All-*trans*-retinoic acid** (induction and maintenance therapy for promyelocytic form, AML M3). **Bone marrow transplant (BMT)** for long-term

survival, age < 60, and poor prognostic patients.

Chronic Myelogenous Leukemia (CML)

1. Common in middle-aged adults. Associated with previous radiation and benzene exposure.
2. Consider CML as a type of leukemia that may occur de novo or secondary to other myeloproliferative disorders and can progress into acute phase (blast crisis) after being stable for years.
3. Findings: Fever, anorexia/weight loss, fatigue, **splenomegaly (usually with blast crisis)**, and night sweats.
4. Diagnosis: CBC (**increased WBCs/leukocytosis**); peripheral smear (**increased WBCs with myeloid cells and basophilia**, and **decreased LAP**. Confirm with **t(9;22) Philadelphia chromosome bcr-abl gene** by karyotyping, fluorescent in situ hybridization (FISH), PCR, bone marrow aspirate.
5. Treatment: **Imatinib mesylate (Gleevec)** by inhibiting bcr-abl tyrosine kinase gene. **Bone marrow transplant (allogeneic)** for long-term survival.

Chronic Lymphocytic Leukemia (CLL)

1. Common in adults > 50 years old. Usually asymptomatic, but may be symptomatic too.
2. Findings: **Lymphadenopathy**, hepatosplenomegaly, fatigue, and **lymphocytosis** (usually incidental finding).
3. Diagnosis: CBC (**Lymphocytosis**); peripheral blood smear (lymphocytes & **smudge cells**); bone marrow biopsy (confirms infiltration with mature lymphocytes). T-cell marker (CD5+).
4. Treatment: **Fludarabine**. Anemia and thrombocytopenia = poor prognosis. No treatment is recommended for asymptomatic patients.
5. *****CLL is related to autoimmune hemolytic anemia.

Hodgkin's Lymphoma

1. A type of cancer that mostly affects young adults. It involves the malignancy of

Reed-Sternberg (RS) cells.

2. Findings: Painless lymph node enlargement (cervical lymphadenopathy), hepatosplenomegaly, fever, night sweats, and weight loss.
3. Diagnosis: Lymph node excisional biopsy (presence of RS cells = owl's eye nuclei); chest CT scan, abdominal/pelvic CT scan, bone marrow biopsies and aspirates.
4. Treatment: Chemotherapy cocktail of doxorubicin, bleomycin, vinblastine, and dacarbazine (ABVD cocktail) +/- radiation therapy.
5. Risk of secondary tumors: breast, lung, colon, thyroid, and bone cancers.

Non-Hodgkin's Lymphoma

1. Can affect any age group.
2. Associated with EBV (Burkitt's lymphoma), HIV/AIDS (CNS B-cell lymphoma), HTLV (T-cell lymphoma), and *H. Pylori* (gastric MALToma).
3. Findings: Lymphadenopathy draining Waldeyer's ring; abdominal, mediastinal, and extranodal involvement; may have chest pains (from lung tumor).
4. Diagnosis: Lymph node biopsy (diffuse small cleaved cells).
5. Treatment: Combination chemotherapy +/- radiation therapy. May add monoclonal antibody anti-CD20 (rituximab).
6. Complications: HIV (CNS lymphoma; treat with anti-retroviral therapy, HAART); tumor lysis syndrome, and gastric MALTomas.

Multiple Myeloma

1. Due to malignancy involving bone marrow's plasma cells and increased production of immunoglobulin heavy/light chains.
2. Findings: Hypercalcemic symptoms ("stones, bones, abdominal moans, and psychiatric overtones"), back pains, fatigue, constipation, fractures, and infections.
3. Diagnosis: **UPEP** (reveals Bence Jones protein), **SPEP,** IgG > 3g/dL. Increased **calcium**, BUN/Cr, hemoglobin (anemia), peripheral blood smear shows "rouleaux" appearance, **full-body skeletal survey with plain radiographs** (punched-out **osteolytic** lesions)**, bone marrow aspirate** (plasma cells > 10%), and **normal LAP levels.**
4. Treatment: Chemotherapy => **melphalan + steroids** +/- thalidomide, **stem cell transplant**. Treatment for the symptoms are: **IVFs, glucocorticoids, diuresis (furosemide)** for hypercalcemia; **bisphosphonates (alendronate) & local radiation** for bone pain/fractures; **IVFs** for renal failure, **erythropoietin** for anemia, and **vaccinate** to prevent infections.
5. Beta-microglobulin is the prognostic factor.

6. **MGUS:** M-protein < 3 g/dL → bone marrow plasma cells < 10% → **normal labs** (hemoglobin, calcium, creatinine) → **normal bone x-ray** → treat with observation. May progress to multiple myeloma.
7. **Solitary plasmacytoma:** single lytic lesion on bone x-ray → all other labs normal → **treat with excision + radiation**. May progress to multiple myeloma.

Lung Cancer

1. The number one cause of cancer mortality.
2. Etiologies: Chronic use of tobacco, asbestos and radon exposures, and second-hand smoking.
3. Findings: Hemoptysis, weight loss, chronic cough, pneumonia, hypercalcemia (mostly squamous cell carcinoma), hoarseness.
4. Diagnosis: Sputum cytology, chest x-ray, CT scan with biopsy or bronchoscopy. Biopsy all palpable lymph nodes first before obtaining chest x-rays. **PET Scans** for large mediastinal lymph nodes and mediastinoscopy for staging. Also obtain abdominal and chest CT scans, bone scan; and CT and MRI of the head for further staging.
5. Treatment: Surgery (non-small cell cancer) and chemotherapy (small-cell cancer). Chemotherapy + radiation for supraclavicular or mediastinal lymphadenopathy, or pleural invasion.
6. Complications: **Pancoast's syndrome** (shoulder pain + Horner's syndrome), **superior vena cava syndrome** (swelling of the face + arm, increased JVP), hoarseness (vocal cord paralysis due to recurrent laryngeal nerve), diaphragm paralysis (phrenic nerve involvement), hypercalcemia (production of parathyroid hormone by squamous cell carcinoma), trousseau's syndrome (hypercoagulable state), hyponatremia/SIADH (due to ADH production by small-cell carcinoma), cushing's syndrome (due to production of adrenocorticotropic hormone, ACTH by small-cell carcinoma), and Eaton-lambert syndrome (muscle fatigue improves with repeated stimulation).
7. **Solitary pulmonary nodule:** Usually benign if nodule is stable for more than 2 years → compare chest x-ray with previous x-rays → if there is no old films, a lung nodule in a smoker or > 35 years old should be evaluated with CT scan. Biopsy may be done for tissue diagnosis. Consider hamartoma or infection (tuberculosis, fungi) when cancer is least suspected → manage with observation/follow-up and chest x-ray/CT scan.

Breast Cancer

1. Risk factors: Prior history of breast cancer (**biggest risk**), older age, family history in first-degree relatives, female gender, early menarche, late menopause,

late first full-term pregnancy, history of atypical hyperplasia, radiation exposure before age 30, obesity, and use of hormone replacement therapy for > 5 years.

2. Findings: **A breast mass found in post-menopausal woman is breast cancer until proven otherwise**. Breast mass can be hard/firm, immobile, painless. Skin changes include ulcer, discharge, erythema, dimpling with axillary lymphadenopathy. Mass usually is at the **upper outer quadrant**.

3. Diagnosis: Initially, palpable breast mass may be present → may proceed with a clinical decision to biopsy. **Mammogram** may be used initially as well. Look for features (microcalcifications, irregular borders, and hyperdense regions). **Suspicious mammogram** should be evaluated with biopsy. **Negative mammogram** should be evaluated further with **ultrasound** (cysts/solid masses), **FNA** (palpable lumps), **stereotactic core biopsy** (non-palpable lumps), or excisional biopsy. Test biopsied samples for **estrogen/progesterone receptors (ER/PR)** and **HER2.**

4. Treatment: Intraductal carcinoma (DCIS) → treat with **mastectomy or wide excision +/- radiation.** Lobular carcinoma in situ (LCIS) → treat with **mastectomy or tamoxifen.** For **invasive ductal carcinoma** → treat with **breast conservation therapy or modified radical mastectomy + radiation therapy**. Treat positive axillary lymph nodes involvement with chemotherapy (**5-FU, methotrexate, doxorubicin, or cyclophosphamide**). Treat ER+ or PR+ malignancies with tamoxifen or raloxifene, and HER2+ with **trastuzumab.**

5. Test genetically high-risk patients for BRCA-1 and BRCA-2.

6. **Fibroadenoma:** women < 30 years of age → round, rubbery, and freely movable → unlikely to be cancer → observe with any changes to menstrual cycles → sometimes, may need biopsy.

7. **Inflammatory cancer of the breast: Poor prognosis,** fast-growing, aggressive, invades lymphatics causing inflammatory skin changes (red, hot skin; may appear similar to mastitis).

8. **Paget's disease of the breast:** Unilateral scaling erosion of the nipple → may cause ductal carcinoma in situ (DCIS) of the nipple and areolar + itching + burning + erosion and ulceration + erythematous + oozing → associated with invasive ductal carcinoma → diagnosis: biopsy of the skin area.

Colorectal Cancer

1. Risk factors: Age (after age 40), family history, and inflammatory bowel disease (ulcerative colitis > Crohn's disease).

2. Findings: May be asymptomatic, bright red blood per rectum (BRBPR), melena, guaiac-positive stool, change in bowel habits, weight loss, fatigue, and anemia (iron deficiency).

3. Diagnosis: Initially, may be palpable mass upon digital rectal exam, **positive fecal occult blood test (FOBT)**, flexible sigmoidoscopy, barium enema, and colonoscopy with biopsy of lesions. **Colonoscopy** is mostly used. **Positive**

occult blood in any patient > 40 years of age is considered colon cancer until proven otherwise.

4. Treatment: Primary surgical resection of involved bowel segment with adjacent mesentery and regional lymph nodes. **5-FU + leucovorin or levamisole** are used as adjuvant chemotherapy. Most common metastasis is to the liver **(poor prognosis)** → treat with chemotherapy or radiofrequency ablation therapy. Solitary metastasis is treated with resection.

5. Family history with colon, ovarian, and endometrial cancer may indicate presence of hereditary nonpolyposis colorectal cancer (HNPCC) in a patient with cancer of the colon.

6. Therefore, screen a patient with family history of polyps or colorectal cancer when the patient is 10 years younger than the affected patient at the time of diagnosis.

7. **Complication: large bowel obstruction.**

Pancreatic Cancer

1. A malignancy of the pancreas. It is considered a ductal adenocarcinoma. It is seen in adults > 50 years of age → mostly at the head of the pancreas.

2. Risk factors: Smoking, chronic pancreatitis, diabetes mellitus.

3. Findings: weight loss, **painless jaundice**, anorexia, epigastric pain, nausea. May present with **migratory thrombophlebitis (Trousseau syndrome)**, **palpable, non-tender gallbladder (Courvoisier sign)**, and venous thromboembolism.

4. Diagnosis: Increased bilirubin, increased aminotransferases, anemia, **abdominal ultrasound** (usually used first), and abdominal/pelvic CT scan.

5. Treatment: Whipple procedure (pancreaticoduodenectomy) if resectable → risk with procedure => **delayed gastric emptying**. If unresectable, treat with chemotherapy or radiation (palliative care only).

6. Associated with **CA 19-9 marker.**

Hepatocellular Cancer

1. Risk factors: Alcohol, viral hepatitis (hepatitis B or C), hemachromatosis, aflatoxin, alpha1-antitrypsin deficiency.

2. Findings: RUQ abdominal pain, jaundice, malaise, fatigue, and weight loss.

3. Diagnosis: Increased aminotransferases, increased bilirubin, and coagulopathy. **Alpha-fetoprotein (AFP)** may be elevated and measured post-operative to detect recurrences. CT scan can be used for diagnostic imaging.

4. Treatment: Surgical resection and liver transplant.

5. **Other tumors of the liver: Hemangioma** => most common primary tumor of the

liver → benign & observe; may require surgery if symptomatic. **Hepatic adenoma** => benign; associated with **OCPs (birth control pills)** → stop OCP pills & observe; may require surgery if symptomatic.

Esophageal Cancer

1. Etiology: **Chronic Barrett's esophageal disorder (metaplasia)**, smoking, and alcohol. The most common type is adenocarcinoma.
2. Findings: Dysphagia, weight loss, anemia, and complaint of 'sticky food.'
3. Diagnosis: Barium swallow and **EGD with biopsy (confirms)**.
4. Treatment: Resection (localized tumor) and chemotherapy + radiation therapy (advanced tumor).

Thyroid Cancer

1. Malignancy of the thyroid gland. Associated with **childhood radiation exposure, multiple endocrine neoplasia (MEN II).**
2. Findings: Firm/hard nodule.
3. Diagnosis: Thyroid Stimulating Hormone (TSH), ultrasound (cold nodule), FNA, or open biopsy, and **increased calcitonin levels.**
4. Treatment: Thyroidectomy.

Prostate Cancer

1. Malignancy of the prostate that affects mostly male adults greater than 80 years of age.
2. Findings: It is known to present as asymptomatic and discovered incidentally during a routine visit and digital rectal examination. Benign prostatic hyperplasia (BPH) symptoms (dysuria + hesistancy + frequency), hematuria, back pain (from vertebral metastases and **osteoblastic lesions**).
3. Diagnosis: Digital rectal exam (DRE) → prostate irregularities or nodules on rectal exam, prostate-specific antigen (PSA), and acid phosphatase. **Ultrasound-guided needle biopsy** may be used for diagnosis and staging.
4. Treatment: **Prostectomy or radiation therapy (brachytherapy or external beam)** for negative nodes; and **androgen ablation & chemotherapy (GnRH agonist-leuprolide, orchiectomy, flutamide, estrogen-diethylstilbesterol, cyproterone)** for positive nodes and metastases. Radiation therapy is used for bone pain/metastases. Elderly patients with low Gleason score may only

require watchful waiting/observation.
5. Gleason score predicts tumor biology → score of 2-10 → from a low to high score means from well-differentiated to poorly-differentiated.

Testicular Cancer

1. Germ cell tumors (e.g. seminoma, nonseminoma) → most common solid malignancies in men < 30 years of age.
2. Risk factors: Observe for **Cryptorchid testis** (cryptorchidism) and Klinefelter's syndrome.
3. Findings: Unilateral scrotal mass.
4. Diagnosis: **Alpha fetoprotein (AFP), beta HCG**, LDH, CT scan of chest/abdomen and pelvis, and radical inguinal orchiectomy (both diagnostic & therapeutic).
5. Treatment: **Radical inguinal orchiectomy with or without chemotherapy or radiation therapy.**

Bladder Cancer

1. Transitional cell carcinoma is the most common cancer of the urinary tract.
2. Associated with smokers, aniline (rubber) dye exposure, and prolonged infection of the urinary tract with *schistosomiasis*.
3. Findings: **Persistent painless hematuria**, dysuria, frequency, and urgency.
4. Diagnosis: Urinary analysis, cytology (dysplastic cells), CT scan with contrast, intravenous pyelogram, and **cystoscopy with biopsy (diagnostic)**.
5. Treatment: Surgery +/- radiation therapy and chemotherapy for metastases.

Ovarian Cancer

1. Asymptomatic initially and presents late in postmenopausal women. This is an epithelial tumor. Most are adenocarcinomas.
2. Risk factors: Age, family history of cancers with BRCA-1, BRCA-2. OCPs are protective factors.
3. Findings: Pelvic mass + ascites + pleural effusion + ovarian enlargement + weight loss + abdominal pain + constipation + bloating + pelvic pressure + urinary frequency +/- vaginal bleeding. An **ovarian mass is a postmenopausal woman is ovarian cancer until proven otherwise.**
4. Diagnosis: Pelvic ultrasound, pelvis CT scan, or MRI; **chest x-ray** (rule out

pleural effusion), and **CA-125 marker**.

5. Treatment: **Debulking surgery with TAH-BSO & omentectomy +** chemotherapy.
6. Complication: **Bowel obstruction** and overall poor prognosis.
7. **Serous cystadenocarcinoma =>** most common type of ovarian cancer + **psammoma bodies.**
8. **Meigs syndrome =>** ovarian fibroma + ascites + right hydrothorax.
9. **Krukenberg tumor =>** stomach cancer with metastases to ovaries.

Uterine Cancer

1. **Postmenopausal vaginal bleeding or uterine bleeding is cancer until proven otherwise →** most common type is endometrial adenocarcinoma.
2. Risk factors: Chronic unopposed estrogen stimulation, late menopause, nulliparity, diabetes mellitus, obesity, hypertension, and hormone (estrogen) replacement therapy.
3. Diagnosis: Endometrial biopsy.
4. Treatment: Surgery +/- radiation therapy.

Cervical Cancer

1. Pap smear screenings decrease incidence and mortality.
2. Risk factors: Human papillomavirus (HPV) infection, multiple sex partners, age < 20 years old with early sexual activity, smoking, low-socioeconomic status with high-risk sexual practices (HIV & other STDs).
3. Findings: **Vaginal bleeding, postcoital bleeding,** vaginal discharge, and pelvic pain.
4. Diagnosis: Colposcopy with biopsy from an abnormal pap smear as **invasive cervical carcinoma or cervical intraepithelial neoplasia (CIN).**
5. Treatment: **CIN I (mild dysplasia)** or **low-grade squamous intraepithelial lesion (LGSIL): treat with observation, pap smear and colposcopy follow-ups every 3-6 months for 1 year.** CIN II/III: treat with **cryosurgery,** laser surgery, conization, or LEEP. Invasive carcinoma: treat with hysterectomy + lymph node dissection. Metastases would require chemotherapy +/- radiation therapy.
6. HPV vaccine, recently approved by FDA, may help to reduce the risk of cervical cancer.

Basal Cell Carcinoma

1. It is associated with the sun and causes the most common skin malignancy.
2. Findings: **Pink pearly papule** usually on the **face** but may be anywhere. Involves sun exposure. **Rodent ulcers.**
3. Diagnosis: Biopsy of lesion (palisading cells with retraction).
4. Treatment: **Surgical excision or MOHs' micrographic surgery +/-** radiation. Other treatments are curettage and cryosurgery.

Malignant Melanoma

1. Known to be the leading cause of death from a dermatological disease.
2. Risk factors: Sun exposure, blue eyes, fair skin, family history, and dysplastic nevi.
3. Findings: Hyperpigmented skin lesion with recent change in size (larger) and appearance (darker and irregular borders).
4. Description of skin lesions indicating high risk for skin carcinoma: => **A** = **A**symmetry, **B** = **B**order (irregular), **C** = **C**olor (dark/variations), **D** = **D**iameter (> 6mm), **E** = **E**levation with surface irregularity.
5. Diagnosis: Biopsy of skin (melanocytes with cellular atypia).
6. Treatment: **Surgical excision** +/- lymph node dissection. Chemotherapy for metastases.
7. **Superficial spreading melanoma** => better prognosis than nodular melanoma (vertically spread = depth). **Prognosis is based on depth.**

Squamous Cell Carcinoma

1. Risk factors: It is related to sun exposure, previous medical history of actinic keratosis, arsenic exposure, radiation, and immunosuppression.
2. Findings: Red exophytic nodules with scaling usually on the **lower lip**.
3. Diagnosis: Biopsy of lesion. Squamous cell carcinoma **in situ => Bowen disease.**
4. Treatment: If biopsy is suspicious, treat with **surgical excision of lesion. MOHs' micrographic surgery +/-** radiation.

Meningioma

1. Brain tumor → usually asymptomatic.

2. Findings: Incidental finding, seizures, neurologic deficits, or signs of intracranial hypertension (headache, nausea, vomiting, blurred vision, papilledema).
3. Diagnosis: CT scan of the head (shows **calcification**).
4. Treatment: **Observe with serial CT scans of the head** if small or asymptomatic, **surgical excision** for larger lesions presenting with symptoms +/- radiation and chemotherapy.

Glioma

1. Findings: Watch for a patient who complains of **awakening headaches from sleep**, nausea and vomiting.
2. Diagnosis: CT scan of the head, MRI, and biopsy for definitive diagnosis.
3. Treatment: Surgical resection + external beam radiation or chemotherapy.
4. Types of glial tumors are astrocytomas, ependymomas, oligodendrogliomas, and mixed gliomas.
5. **Glioblastoma multiforme** => a serious brain tumor that appears on CT scan as unifocal and centrally necrotic enhancing lesion. Look for edema and mass effect around the lesion.

ONCOLOGY 1-LINER JUNKY CASES

- Cord compression → start **emergency corticosteroids**; then obtain MRI → follow with radiation therapy → then surgical decompression.
- Give ALL patients **allopurinol** before chemotherapy to prevent **tumor lysis syndrome**.
- Tumor lysis syndrome => hyperkalemia + hyperphosphatemia + hyperuricemia + hypocalcemia → treat with vigorous hydration + allopurinol.
- Treat neutropenia → with recombinant human hematopoietic growth factors (G-CSF or GM-CSF).
- Leukemoid reactions → leukocytosis due to infection, inflammation, stress, and malignancies.
- Hairy cell leukemia => malignancy of B lymphocytes → peripheral blood smear: **hairy cytoplasmic projections + CD11c positivity** → bone marrow biopsy: "dry bone marrow tap."
- CML → associated with increased **vitamin B12**.
- Mycosis fungoides/Sezary syndrome => peripheral blood smear: cerebriform nuclei "butt cells" → plaque patches skin lesions → difficult to treat → pautrier abscesses in skin.
- Burkitt lymphoma => common in African children with Epstein-Barr virus.
- **Waldenstrom's macroglobulinemia** => increased IgM + hyperviscosity syndrome → symptoms include headache, chest pains, blurred vision, papilledema → treat hyperviscosity with emergency plasmapheresis; may also use alkylating agents: chlorambucil + prednisone, cyclophosphamide, melphalan, CHOP; others: fludarabine or 2-CdA → related to cold agglutinins.
- Myelodysplasia/myelofibrosis => associated with CML → bone marrow biopsy shows "dry tap" → anemia + high mean corpuscular volume (MCV) & red cell distribution index.
- **Metastatic** cancer of the liver → most common malignancy of the liver.
- Pancoast's syndrome => shoulder pain + lower brachial plexopathy + Horner's syndrome (miosis, ptosis, anhidrosis) → due to invasion of cervical sympathetic chain.
- Eaton-Lambert syndrome => muscle fatigue improves with repeated stimulation.
- Superior vena cava syndrome => elevated JVP + right-sided swelling of face + arm → treat with radiation therapy.
- Trousseau's syndrome => hypercoagulable state with adenocarcinoma.
- Cholangiosarcoma => associated with IBD (ulcerative colitis), liver flukes (*Clonorchis* spp.) increase risk in immigrants.
- Angiosarcoma => associated with vinyl chloride exposure.
- Hepatoblastoma => primary tumor of the liver in children.
- Gastric adenocarcinoma => Asian adults > 50 years of age → iron deficiency

anemia → confirm with EGD and biopsy → treat with surgical resection or radiation therapy + chemotherapy.

- Carcinoid tumors => affects the appendix or small bowel → carcinoid syndrome: associated with **serotonin** → causes flushing + abdominal pain + diarrhea + tricuspid regurgitation → diagnose with **increased 5-HIAA or chromogranin A** → treat with surgical resection + **octreotide.**

- Craniopharyngioma => in children → **remnant of rathke pouch** → **highly calcified lesions** around pineal gland @ region of sella turcica → leads to bitemporal hemianopia.

- Watch pseudotumor cerebri → benign tumor → **obese patient** + papilledema + headaches + vomiting + negative CT/MRI scans → diagnose with lumbar puncture abnormality only (**high pressure**) → treat with weight loss or underlying illness → **repeat lumbar punctures** may help to lower intracranial pressure and with ocular problems.

- Histiocytosis => **birbeck granules** (cytoplasmic inclusion bodies similar to tennis rackets) → CD1-positive histiocyte (malignant cell).

Chapter 7
Pulmonology
Asthma

1. This is usually a childhood illness consisting of 'atopic triad' such as eczema, seasonal rhinitis, and wheezing.
2. Etiology: It leads to chronic inflammatory process involving the airway tracts.
3. Findings: May be seasonal; shortness of breath with chest tightness, intermittent wheezing, and coughing. Evaluate any difficulty to speak, cyanosis, or use of accessory muscles to determine the severity of asthma attack. Wheezing may be present, indicating severe exacerbation.
4. Diagnosis: **PFTs** indicating **obstruction** with decreased ratio of forced expiratory volume in 1 second (FEV1) to forced vital capacity (FVC); which is usually reversible with **bronchodilators (albuterol)** by 12%. Obtain **ABG**, chest x-ray, and methacholine challenge test.
5. Treatment: **Acute asthma** => Albuterol (short-acting beta-2 agonist, bronchodilator), inhaled corticosteroids, and systemic corticosteroids (methylprednisolone or prednisone); **chronic asthma** => depending on the symptoms, include PRN short-acting bronchodilator, low- to medium-dose inhaled corticosteroids, long-acting bronchodilator, high-dose inhaled corticosteroids, and systemic steroids.
6. Additional treatment for prophylaxis or chronic cases may include cromolyn and zafirlukast. Theophylline, a phosphodiesterase inhibitor, may be used in cases where other agents show no response.
7. Avoid triggers including advising the parents of patients to stop smoking.

Emphysema/Chronic Obstructive Pulmonary Disease (COPD)

1. Etiology: Destruction of lung parenchyma leading to **decreased elastic recoil and air trapping**.
2. Associated with **chronic smoking history**.
3. Findings: Cough, wheezing, shortness of breath (dyspnea), some may have barrel chest +/- weight loss and clubbing of the fingers.
4. Diagnosis: PFTs, **decreased FEV1/FVC ratio < 0.75-0.80** (less than 75%-80%), chest x-ray (hyperinflated and flat diaphragms).
5. Treatment: **Acute COPD** (exacerbations with increased dyspnea & change in

cough or sputum production) => screen with chest x-ray for cause, **oxygen** should be maintained around 90%, **albuterol** (inhaled beta agonist, bronchodilator), **ipratropium** (anti-cholinergics), **systemic corticosteroids,** and antibiotics (azithromycin, TMP-SMX, amoxicillin) as needed. **Chronic COPD** => oxygen should be given when room air SaO2 < 88% or PaO2 < 55 mmHg (and in **cor pulmonale**), **albuterol** (inhaled beta agonist, bronchodilator), and **ipratropium** (anti-cholinergics). Long-term **oxygen** therapy and **smoking cessation reduce mortality**. **Pulmonary rehabilitation** is considered a long-term benefit.
6. Complication: **Cor pulmonale** as a result of right heart failure from pulmonary hypertension.
7. Give patients annual **influenza** and **pneumococcal vaccinations**.

Pneumonia

1. Etiology: *Streptococcus Pneumoniae* infection in ages > 40 years old.
2. Findings: Fever > 102 °F, malaise, shortness of breath, hypoxia, cough, and sputum production.
3. Diagnosis: Chest x-ray, **sputum gram stain** and **culture**, ABG, and pulse oximeter.
4. Treatment: oxygen, IV fluoroquinolone (inpatient) or third-generation cephalosporin and azithromycin. Azithromycin can also be used as outpatient.

Pulmonary Embolus

1. Etiology: Deep venous thrombosis (DVT), immobility, trauma, surgery, pregnancy, recent fracture, use of birth control pills (OCPs), obesity, CHF, coagulation abnormalities, and malignancies.
2. Findings: Dyspnea in a DVT patient, unilateral leg pain +/- swelling, tachycardia, tachypnea, chest pain, a loud P2 or S2, and increased JVP. Hypotension and shock may be seen too.
3. Diagnosis: **ABG** (respiratory alkalosis, increased A-a gradient), **chest x-ray (may be normal)**, ECG (S wave in lead I, Q wave in lead III, T wave in lead III), **V/Q scan** (based on the pretest probability; if intermediate, should be **confirmed with CT angiography**), and **pulmonary angiography** (gold standard).
4. Treatment: IV heparin or LMWH, warfarin (target INR to 2.0-3.0), tPA (with heparin for hypotension/shock), and IVC filter. Treat first-time thrombotic patients for 3-6 months and life-long treatment in recurrent patients or if positive antiphospholipid syndrome, prosthetic heart valves, and recurrent DVTs or PEs).

Pneumothorax

1. Air in the pleural space.
2. Etiology: Iatrogenic, traumatic, or spontaneous. Watch for history of COPD, cystic fibrosis, trauma, and central lines that predispose patients to pneumothorax.
3. Findings: Dyspnea, pleuritic chest pain, decreased breath sounds and tactile fremitus, tympany on percussion on same side, and +/- tracheal deviation **toward** the affected side.
4. Diagnosis: Chest x-ray (observe for collapse and tracheal deviation).
5. Treatment: **Chest tube insertion**, oxygen, morphine or NSAIDs. A smaller pneumothorax is managed supportively with oxygen and observation. Treat recurrent pneumothorax with **pleurodesis**.

- **Tension Pneumothorax**: Etiology: Penetrating trauma, COPD, or positive end-expiratory pressure (PEEP). **Findings:** Presents as pneumothorax but with **hypotension, increased JVP, shock**, absent breath sounds, hypertympanic, or hyperresonant percussion sound on the affected side. **Diagnosis:** Chest x-ray (tracheal deviation **away** from the affected side). **Treatment: Emergency needle thoracentesis** (for decompression; placed at the anterior second intercostal space), then **chest or thoracostomy tube** insertion.

Pleural Effusion

1. Fluid in the pleural space → classified as transudative or exudative per pleural fluid diagnostic.
2. Etiology: Congestive heart failure (CHF), malignancy, or pneumonia.
3. Findings: Pleuritic chest pain, decreased breath sounds, decreased tactile fremitus, and dullness to percussion on the affected side.
4. Diagnosis: **Thoracentesis** (diagnostic & therapeutic) and obtain WBCs, cell count with differential, serum LDH, total & serum protein, pH, acid-fast bacilli, gram stain and culture, glucose and triglycerides. From the thoracentesis analysis, **transudative** shows pleural/serum protein ratio of less than 0.5, pleural/serum LDH ratio of less than 0.6, and pleural LDH less than 200; while **exudative** shows pleural/serum protein ratio of greater than 0.5, pleural/serum LDH ratio of greater than 0.6, and pleural LDH greater than 200.
5. Treatment: **Thoracentesis**. Insert a **chest tube** into the pleural space if pH < 7.2, WBCs > 100,000, or glucose < 40 (indicates **empyema**). Malignant pleural fluid must be sent in for cytology. Pleurodesis and decortication may be used if recurrent or there's no response to therapy.
6. Complications: **Empyema** (pus); **pneumothorax & bleeding** (from procedural thoracentesis).

Acute Respiratory Distress Syndrome (ARDS)

1. Inflammation of the lung parenchyma which leads to noncardiogenic pulmonary edema and alveolar damage → usually due to an underlying illness.
2. Etiology: Sepsis, trauma, ICU, burn, pancreatitis, pneumonia, drug overdose, blood transfusion, near drowning, and shock.
3. Findings: **Difficult to oxygenate hypoxia**, rales/rhonchi, cyanosis, and intercostal retractions. ARDS occurs with 24-48 hours of the initial insult.
4. Diagnosis: Usually diagnosed with difficulty to oxygenate hypoxic patient despite maximal oxygen administration, **chest x-ray (diffuse bilateral pulmonary infiltrates with pulmonary edema)**, and **PaO2/FiO2 ratio (< 200 is ARDS)**.
5. Treatment: **Intubation + mechanical ventilation** w/high oxygen therapy, **low tidal volumes, positive end-expiratory pressure (PEEP)**, and treat the underlying etiology.

Obstructive Sleep Apnea (OSA)

1. Repetitive occurrence of airway collapse leading to occasional hypoxia and arousal from sleep.
2. Etiology: Obesity, spontaneous.
3. Findings: Obese, fatigue, snoring & apnea (usually complained by spouse), unrefreshing sleep, early morning headaches, excessive daytime sleepiness or difficulty staying up while driving, neck circumference > 17 cm, retrognathia, and large tonsils. Patients may have hypertension.
4. Diagnosis: Sleep study (polysomnography), apnea-hypopnea index (AHI): diagnose if > 5, ABG (chronic respiratory acidosis with chronic metabolic alkalosis compensation).
5. Treatment: Weight loss, **continuous positive airway pressure (CPAP) is most effective**, and surgery such as uvulopalatopharyngoplasty (UPPP) as last resort.
6. Complications: Increased risk of **motor vehicle accidents (MVAs), pulmonary hypertension**, and **diabetes**.
7. For central sleep apnea (from the CNS), treat with acetazolamide or medroxyprogesterone.

Sarcoidosis

1. Etiology: A systemic condition that is idiopathic. It involves multiple organs. It is a diagnosis of exclusion.
2. Findings: Chronic cough, dyspnea, fatigue, weight loss, uveitis, erythema nodosum, and arthritis. Also associated with **negative PPD test**.
3. Diagnosis: PFTs, chest x-ray (**bilateral hilar lymphadenopathy +/- infiltrates**), increased serum calcium and ACE levels, **bronchoalveolar lavage**, and **tissue biopsy of the lung/lymph node** (noncaseating granulomas).
4. Treatment: Corticosteroids (prednisone).

***Solitary pulmonary nodule:** Usually benign if nodule is stable for > 2 years → this is why you compare chest x-ray with previous x-rays → if there is no old films, a lung nodule in a smoker or > 35 years old should be evaluated with CT scan. Biopsy may be done for tissue diagnosis. Consider hamartoma or infection (tuberculosis, fungi) when cancer is least suspected → manage with observation/follow-up and chest x-ray/CT scan.

PULMONOLOGY 1-LINER JUNKY CASES

- Increased TLC => obstruction; decreased TLC => restrictive lung diseases.
- Other causes of wheezing => cystic fibrosis, bronchiolitis, and foreign body → **remember do not automatically assume that when a patient wheezes it is asthma! It could be anything affecting the airway!!**
- Avoid beta blockers in asthmatic and COPD patients!
- **Foreign body aspiration** => sudden, **unilateral**.
- Chronic cough that worsens in supine position (sleeping) => think **GERD**!
- Inhaled corticosteroids are safe during pregnancy.
- Do not treat patients without symptoms → remember asthma in children resolves by early adulthood.
- Use bronchodilators **before exercise** in exercise-induced asthma.
- An asthmatic patient who has stopped hyperventilation and with 'normal' PCO2 (discovered on **ABG**) should be intubated! Upon discharge, peak flow (meter) measurements should be obtained at home.
- COPD => increased total lung capacity (TLC = obstruction) → due to increased residual volume (RV); COPD is irreversible with beta-2 agonist (bronchodilator).
- Chronic bronchitis => classified as three months of productive cough over a two-year period.
- Watch other causes of '**change in chronic cough**' (if **without** sputum production) in a patient → think of **lung cancer**!
- Remember the **50:50 rule** => **intubate** patients with CO2 > 50 mmHg and O2 < 50 mmHg.
- A pleural effusion on chest x-ray with thickness > 10 mm warrants a thoracentesis.
- Foreign body aspiration => occurs usually at the right middle lobe (bronchus) → presents with recurrent pneumonia.
- Alpha1-antitrypsin disorder → autosomal recessive; causes cirrhosis of the liver + emphysema of the lung → diagnosis: chest x-ray, low or absent of alpha1-antitrypsin on serum protein electrophoresis (SPEP), genotype analysis, low albumin and inceased prothrombin time → treat by replacing alpha1-antitrypsin + liver transplantation.

Chapter 8
Infectious Disease
Skin Infections
Impetigo

1. Infection of the superficial layers of the epidermis due to trauma, insect bites, or scabies. This infection is contagious.
2. Etiology: *Streptococcus pyogenes* (**group A, the most common cause**) and *Staphylococcus aureus* (**with presence of furuncle**) bacterial infections.
3. Findings: Erythematous macule → it **changes to vesicle/pustule** (primary lesion) → ruptures & **becomes yellow/honey-colored exudate**.
4. Diagnosis: Culture of the base of the lesion.
5. Treatment: Topical mupirocin, dicloxacillin, or cephalexin.
6. Complication: **Poststreptococcal glomerulonephritis**.

Erysipelas

1. Superficial cellulitis usually due to *streptococcus pyogenes* (**group A**) bacterial infections from trauma or breaks in the skin. Affects the dermis and epidermis layers.
2. Findings: **Bright red, very painful & tender on palpation, shiny**, and **edematous** lesion or plaque usually on the face or extremities.
3. Diagnosis: Culture of the lesion.
4. Treatment: Penicillin.

Soft Tissue Infections
Cellulitis

1. Infection of the dermis involving **subcutaneous tissues**.
2. Etiology: *Streptococcus pyogenes* (**group A, most common cause**) and *Staphylococcus aureus* bacterial infections. Associated with a break in the skin (*S. pyogenes*), bites (*Pasteurella, Eikenella,* anaerobes), or as ulcers and abscess (*S. Aureus*); all defined as the identifiable portal of entry.
3. Findings: Erythematous, warm/heat, swollen, with localized pain/tenderness.

There is occasional fever, chills, and lymphangitis (red streaks).

4. Diagnosis: Usually a clinical diagnosis. Obtain **CBC**, **blood cultures**, and **x-rays** as needed to rule out necrotizing fasciitis.

5. Treatment: Demarcate/mark borders and treat with antistaphylococcal penicillin (**oxacillin**), 2nd generation (**cefazolin**) or 1st generation cephalosporin (**cephalexin**). If allergic to penicillin, treat with **clindamycin**. If MRSA is suspected, consider doxycycline, bactrim, quinolone, but with **severe MRSA use vancomycin**. If there is resistant to vancomycin, use **linezolid**. (Remember treat empirically, **patients with MRSA risk factors**: recent antibiotic use, diabetic, previous MRSA infection or colonization, recent hospitalization, hemodialysis, or IV drug abuser).

6. **Other infections of cellulitis**: *Pseudomonas* spp (diabetic with foot ulcers) treat with antipseudomonal coverage; *pastuerella multocida* (from cat or dog bites) treat with ampicillin or amoxicillin-clavulanate; *vibro vulnificus* (fishermen or salt-water exposure) treat with tetracycline.

Necrotizing Fasciitis

1. **Complication of cellulitis** leading to life-threatening infection of the fascia and soft tissues extending rapidly along **fascial planes and via veins** and **lymphatics**.

2. Etiology: *Streptococcus pyogenes* (**group A,** with skin infections), *Clostridium perfringens* (with gas gangrene), and multiple organisms such as **mixed aerobic** and **anaerobic bacteria** from the GI system.

3. Findings: Pain, systemic toxicity with fever, tenderness, tachycardia, hypotension, decreased [strength, pulses, and sensation], and cutaneous findings such as erythema, bulla, necrosis, gangrene, crepitus, and rapid, dark skin discoloration.

4. Diagnosis: **Clinical diagnosis is challenging**; obtain **radiographs, CT scan, or MRI** to **evaluate for gas and soft tissue** involvement. However, **surgical exploration may be required early in diagnosis**.

5. Treatment: Penicillin (*S. Pyogenes)* with clindamycin (shuts down toxin production), vancomycin (MRSA coverage), and piperacillin/tazobactam (aerobic & anaerobic). **Surgical exploration/surgical fasciotomy** (obtain consult for debridement and fasciotomy) is **critical in diagnosis and treatment**.

6. **Complications: Compartment syndrome** (if delay in diagnosis), **streptococcal toxic shock syndrome** (caused by exotoxin, acts as superantigen), multi-organ failure, and eventually death.

Osteomyelitis

1. A serious bone infection that occurs as a result of hematogenous spread or direct entry from a wound or an adjacent site of infection.

2. Involves the metaphyses of long bones in children including tibia, femur, humerus, and the adult vertebrae.
3. Etiology: *Staphylococcus aureus* (**most common cause**). Others are *salmonella* (most common in sickle cell patients), *Escherichia coli*), *Pseudomonas* (in IV drug user)*, Serratia,* and polymicrobial (gram-negative and anaerobic bacteria are usually the cause in diabetic foot ulcers).
4. Findings: Pain with erythema, tenderness, and edema with occasional fever, chills, and ulcer of the skin.
5. Diagnosis: Obtain initially, radiographs (plain films, but it **may not become positive until 10 days later**), and CT scan, bone scan, or MRI may be positive as **early as 2 days**. However, **bone biopsy with culture is the definite means of diagnosis**.
6. Treatment: If not septic, obtain specimen from **surgical debridement**, then **initiate broad-spectrum coverage** of antimicrobial therapy for possible organisms until the exact organism has been identified with sensitivity. IV antibiotic treatment is for 4-6 weeks. **If septic, usually within 48 hours with poor response to antibiotic therapy**, surgical debridement should be considered immediately. Vertebral osteomyelitis also requires surgery. For broad-spectrum coverage and gram-positive *S. aureus*, **use oxacillin or cefazolin**; for *Pseudomonas*, **use combination of aminoglycoside** and **gentamicin**.
7. In chronic osteomyelitis, management includes complete drainage, debridement, removal of prosthetic material, and antibiotics.
8. Complications: Chronic osteomyelitis, amputation, sepsis, and death.

Septic Arthritis

1. A serious condition that is caused by a joint infection leading to joint damage.
2. Etiology: Systemic bacterial infection usually from *Staphylococcus aureus*. Risk factors include recent instrumentation, arthroscopy, arthroplasty, or IV drug use.
3. Findings: Warm, edematous, erythematous, and tender joint with **limited range of motion**. Watch for multiple affected joints indicating **gonococcal infection**.
4. Diagnosis: Blood cultures, **arthrocentesis** that includes gram stain, culture, cell count with differential, and crystal presence.
5. Treatment: If not septic, obtain specimen from **aspiration** or **surgical debridement**, then **initiate broad-spectrum coverage** of antimicrobial therapy (**nafcillin**) for possible organisms until the exact organism has been identified with sensitivity. IV antibiotic treatment is for 4-6 weeks.

Sexually Transmitted Diseases

(STDs)
Syphilis

1. Etiology: STD caused by *Treponema pallidum*.
2. Findings: **Primary** => occurs within few weeks after exposure; presents as **painless chancre** that is indurated, raised edges with superficial ulceration. **Secondary**: Within 6 weeks to 18 months of primary infection, patients may present with condyloma lata, maculopapular rash involving the mucosal surfaces, palms and soles, malaise, and diffuse lymphadenopathy. **Tertiary**: Usually occurs years after initial/primary infection. Patients may present with gummas (granulomas) affecting different organs, cardiovascular disease (thoracic aortic aneurysms), and neurological signs and symptoms (paresis, neurosyphilis, dementia, tabes dorsalis, Argyll Robertson pupil, and Charcot joints).
3. Diagnosis: **Darkfield microscopy (for lesions only; shows spirochete)**. For screening, obtain non-treponemal serologic test: Venereal Disease Research Laboratory (VDRL) or rapid plasmin reagin (RPR) test; and obtain **fluorescent treponemal antibody, absorbed test** (**FTA-ABS**) or microhemagglutination-*Treponema pallidum* test (MHA-TP) for **confirmation**.
4. Treatment: Penicillin G. If allergic to penicillin, use erythromycin.
5. Obtain lumbar puncture in HIV patients especially in those positive for at least one year.

Genital Herpes

1. STD usually caused by Herpes simplex virus (HSV) Type 2.
2. Findings: Painful grouped vesicle lesions (contagious) in the genital area. Patients may also present with myalgia, fever, and painful inguinal lymphadenopathy.
3. Diagnosis: Vesicle fluid analysis with viral PCR.
4. Treatment: Topical and per oral acyclovir. Begin treatment as soon as symptoms present.
5. Complication: Recurrences requiring daily or long-term therapy.
6. HSV Type 1 causes oral lesions.

Genital Warts

1. Most common cause of acquired STD; caused by HPV 6 and 11 → abstinence is the key to prevention → contagious on skin contact.

2. Findings: Presents as cauliflower or filiform projections with fusion at the base of lesions.
3. Diagnosis: usually screened with pap smear, cytology, and HPV DNA testing. Start to screen in sexually-active women 3 years after the onset of sexual intercourse or at the age of 21; whichever is earlier.
4. Treatment: imiquimod (aldara), topical podophyllin resin or topical podofilox, and **trichloroacetic acid (preferred in pregnancy**; also is cryotherapy, electrocautery, and surgical excision).
5. Complication: Respiratory papillomatosis during vaginal delivery.

Cervicitis or Urethritis

1. A bacterial-causing infection of the cervix or urethral.
2. Etiology: Caused by chlamydial and gonococcal infections.
3. Findings: In women => purulent vaginal discharge with dysuria and dypareunia. Sometimes, patients may be asymptomatic with only vaginal discharge. In men => purulent penile discharge with dysuria.
4. Diagnosis: Urine PCR for chlamydia and gonorrhea; or endocervical/urethral culture for chlamydia and gonorrhea.
5. Treatment: Treat patients for both infections along with their sexual partners. Azithromycin (chlamydia) and ceftriaxone/ciprofloxacin (gonorrhea).

Pelvic Inflammatory Disease (PID)

1. Defined as infection of the upper genital tract that is usually caused by complication of either chlamydia or gonorrhea infection or both. *E. coli* has also been known to cause PID. *Actinomyces Israeli* is associated with intrauterine device (IUD) use. Therefore, IUD is not recommended once a patient has been diagnosed with an STD.
2. Findings: Fever +/- chills, purulent cervical discharge, dyspareunia, pelvic/abdominal pain, adnexal tenderness and cervical motion tenderness.
3. Diagnosis: CBC with differential (**elevated WBCs**), ESR, gram stain, and endocervical smear.
4. Treatment: For outpatient => use **2nd generation cephalosporin** (cefoxitin) or ceftriaxone, and **doxycycline**. In patient => use clindamycin + gentamicin.
5. Complications: Tubo-ovarian abscess (usually palpable on examination), abscess rupture (**treat with emergent laparotomy**), infertility (scarring of the tubes). Note that PID is the **most common cause of preventable infertility** by using condoms.

Genitourinary Tract Infections
Cystitis

1. Etiology: *E. coli* causes about 80% of uncomplicated UTIs. Other causes are *Proteus, Klebsiella,* and *Enterobacter*.
2. Findings: Dysuria, frequency, urgency, and suprapubic pain.
3. Diagnosis: Based on history, urinary analysis (WBCs, bacteria, leukocyte esterase, **no nitrite**) and urine culture.
4. Treatment: TMP-SMX or fluoroquinolone.

Prostatitis

1. Etiology: Caused by gram-negative bacteria (*E. coli, Klebsiella, Proteus*).
2. Findings: Fever +/- chills, dysuria, extreme prostatic tenderness, perineal discomfort, and low back pain. Tender gland on digital rectal exam.
3. Diagnosis: gram stain and urine culture.
4. Treatment: Fluoroquinolone (ciprofloxacin), TMP-SMX, or third-generation cephalosporin for 7-10 days. For chronic prostatis, treat with fluoroquinolone for 12 weeks.

Pyelonephritis

1. Etiology: Caused by gram-negative bacteria (*E. coli, Klebsiella, Proteus*).
2. Findings: Patients are more ill-appearing; nausea, vomiting, fever, shaking chills, dysuria, **flank pain (CVA tenderness)**, with occasional diarrhea. Other possible symptoms are tachycardia and hypotension.
3. Diagnosis: Check for **bacteria in urine** with **leukocytosis (increased WBCs) WBC casts**, urine +/- blood culture.
4. Treatment: IV Fluoroquinolone.

Tuberculosis

1. Etiology: Caused by tubercle bacilli which upon ingestion, they are transported

into the lymph nodes.

2. Findings: Presents as **primary** (based in middle + lower ,lungs with lymphadenopathy; usually heal spontaneously & evolve to small calcified nodule known as Ghon complex), **latent** (positive PPD test with negative chest x-ray), or **extrapulmonary TB** (may affect any organ in immunocompromised patients).

3. Diagnosis: PPD skin test (screen for prior myobacterial exposure; delayed type hypersensitivity reaction), sputum for acid-fast organisms, and chest x-ray.

4. Treatment: **Rifampin, isoniazid (INH), pyrazinamide**, and **ethambutol** for **two months**, then **rifampin** and **isoniazid alone** for **additional four months**. For patients with only latent TB infection, treat with isoniazid for nine months. Remember to give vitamin B6, pyridoxine, to prevent isoniazid-inducing neuropathy. **HIV patients** may require a substitution of rifampin with **rifabutin** to avoid drug-interaction of rifampin with HAART therapy.

Rabies

1. Etiology: Caused by bites from bats, raccoons, skunks, or foxes; occasional dog bites, but less common due to rabies vaccination.

2. Findings: Hydrophobia, drooling, muscle spasms, and then paralysis. Remember, incubation period is usually 1-2 months.

3. Diagnosis: Direct fluorescent antibody (DFA) test (for the presence of rabies virus antigens in brain tissue of animal), and in humans, samples of saliva, serum and spinal fluid (for antibodies to rabies virus), and skin biopsies.

4. Treatment: Based on the following → all wounds should be **cleaned with soap and water** without any suturing needed. In cases of **cats or dogs, if animal is healthy** and available/captured, **observe** for 10 days. If animal presents with symptoms & the patient was **not previously vaccinated, give rabies vaccine + rabies immune globulin**. If the patient was **already vaccinated**, just **give rabies vaccine alone**. If a **WILD animal** (bat, skunk, raccoon, fox) **is caught**, it should be killed and its tissue examined for rabies; **give at least the rabies vaccine even if patient was already vaccinated!** If the **tissue is positive for rabies, give both rabies vaccine + rabies immune globulin**. If a **wild animal**, as described above, is not caught (**escapes after a bite**), **give rabies vaccine + rabies immune globulin**.

Acute HIV Infection

1. Acute retroviral syndrome occurs in 1-4 weeks of being exposed to HIV. This is seen in 50-90% of patients.

2. Findings: Patients present with symptoms that are flu-like and vague such as low-grade fever, malaise, headache, anorexia, and lymphadenopathy. Other symptoms

which may be seen are weight loss, maculopapular rash of the palms and soles, **oral lesions**, peripheral neuropathy, Guillain-Barre syndrome, radiculopathy, Bell's palsy, cognitive impairment, and meningo-encephalitis.

3. Diagnosis: **HIV ELISA** (may take 2-3 months after exposure to HIV to be positive of antibody) and **confirm with Western blot** in patients with positive ELISA test. Also monitor viral load.

4. Treatment: Initiate treatment (highly active antiretroviral therapy, HAART) in patients with symptoms, CD4 count (< 200) and viral load ($> 50,000$). Treatment usually includes three drugs such as **zidovudine**, nevirapine, and indinavir.

5. Complications: Numerous side effects from multidrug therapy and opportunistic infections which these patients are more prone because of their decreased immune system with the presence of Acquired Immune Deficiency Syndrome (AIDS).

6. **Vaccinations =>** give influenza vaccine annually, pneumococcal vaccine every five years, and hepatitis A and B vaccine to HIV patients with hepatitis C.

INFECTIOUS DISEASE 1-LINER JUNKY CASES

- Patients with recurrent MRSA of soft tissue infections such as cellulitis are considered **nasal carriers** → treat with **mupirocin nasal** to the nares.
- Minor cat and dog bites should be cleaned with sterile or tap water and debridement → however, puncture wounds from cat & **human bites (highest risk of infection)** should be given antibiotic prophylaxis.
- Ecthyma gangrenosum => caused by *P. aeruginosa* → common in critically ill patients (AIDS, malignancy, steroid use) → presents as hemorrhagic pustules that changes to necrotic ulcers with erythema around them → treat with antipseudomonal antibiotic (piperacillin and gentamicin).
- **Vestibular papillae** => flesh-colored, soft, pearly papules that are benign and symmetrically distributed in the inner aspect of labia minora.
- **Molluscum contagiosum** => 'central depression,' umbilicated pearly papules filled with pus → treat with liquid nitrogen → common in immunocompromised patients.
- **Progressive multifocal leucoencephalopathy** => etiology: Papovavirus JC → presents with **dementia**, dysarthria, hemiparesis, aphasia → diagnosis: CT scan or MRI of the head, **CSF analysis for JC virus by PCR (confirms)** → treatment: HAART therapy.
- Herpes Simplex virus (HSV) encephalitis => usually caused by HSV type I reactivation → Findings: neurological such as speech abnormality, hearing impairment, **bizarre behavior**, and gustatory or olfactory hallucinations → diagnosis: **CSF** which includes **HSV PCR and culture** and MRI (for temporal lobe lesions) → treatment: acyclovir.
- West Nile encephalitis => associated with Guillain-Barre syndrome (due to acute flaccid paralysis/fasciculations) → diagnosis: CSF for viral meningitis, and test the CSF by ELISA for IgM antibody to West nile virus or IgG → remember, patients who are immunocompromised (like diabetes, HIV/AIDS) can present with West Nile encephalitis.
- **Pneumocystis carinii pneumonia (PCP)** => HIV patients with CD4 < 200 → Findings: fever, dyspnea, non-productive cough → diagnosis: chest x-ray (shows bilateral interstitial infiltrates, ground-glass type), methenamine silver stain of sputum for PCP or bronchoalveolar lavage for PCP, and LDH (increased) → treatment: IV TMP-SMX or pentamidine. Add prednisone when PaO2 is < 70 mmHg or with an A-a gradient > 35 mmHg.
- **Toxoplasmosis** => HIV patients with CD4 < 100 → Findings: headache, chorioretinitis, encephalitis → diagnosis: serology IgG, CT scan/MRI of the head (ring-enhancing lesion) → treatment: sulfadiazine and pyrimethamine.
- **Cryptococcal meningitis** => AIDS with CD4 < 50 → sign & symptoms: fever, headache, delirium → diagnosis: lumbar puncture, india ink and cryptococcal antigen in serum and CSF → treatment: Amphotericin B + fluconazole.

- **Histoplasmosis** => usually common in immunocompromised patients; associated with Ohio, Mississippi river, and exposure to birds, bat guano → Findings: fever, weight loss, upper respiratory infection, splenomegaly → diagnosis: silver staining and culture of specimen, and test urine and serum for *Histoplasma* antigen → treatment: Amphotericin B and itraconazole.
- **Bacterial meningitis** => presents with headaches, neck stiffness, fever, nausea, vomiting, and photophobia → diagnosis: lumbar puncture → treatment: **do not wait if there is high suspicion**, proceed with broad-spectrum antibiotic → **always obtain a CT scan prior to a lumbar puncture when there are signs of increased intracranial pressure/focal neurologic deficit.**
- Periorbital infections => milder case of orbital infection → may be treated with 1st generation cephalosporin (cephalexin).
- Orbital infections => this is a serious infection of the orbital area → patients present with decreased visual acquity, proptosis, oculomotor abnormalities, and chemosis → diagnosis: blood cultures, CBC, and CT scan → treatment: IV nafcillin (broad-spectrum), then obtain **surgical consultation** → complication: without immediate treatment, may lead to **blindness, meningitis,** and **carvenous sinus thrombosis**.
- **Lyme Disease** => caused by exposure to tick bites → Findings: fever, headache, myalgia, fatigue, arthralgias with presence of **erythema chronicum migrans**, and neurologic symptoms (disseminated) → diagnosis: **usually clinical**; may obtain serology test for disseminated Lyme's disease with ELISA → treatment: doxycycline, ceftriaxone, or amoxicillin (drug of choice in pregnant patients) → prevention is with wearing protective clothing (long sleeves) and insect repellant → complications: bilateral facial palsy and heart block (treat with ceftriaxone).
- **Rocky Mountain spotted fever** => rashes on wrists and ankles → treatment: doxycycline or chloramphenicol in pregnant patients.
- **Febrile Neutropenia** => in the case of absolute neutropenia < 500, start **neupogen, cefepime** (to cover gram-negative bacteria) → if MRSA is suspected, start **vancomycin** → and if there's still no response after 48 hours, start **amphotericin B** (antifungal).
- Pharyngitis => usually caused by viral infection (rhinovirus/adenovirus), but bacteria are also known to be involved such as *Streptococcus* (group A) → Findings: fever, sore throat, cough, painful cervical lymphadenopathy, and tonsillar exudates → diagnosis: rapid antigen test for streptococcal infection + throat swab for culture → treatment: **penicillin** & eradicate chronic carriers of positive throat culture with clindamydin.
- Acute sinusitis => usually caused by viral infection (most common cause); however bacterial infection (*S. pneumonia, H. influenza,* and *M. catarrhalis*) can be the cause too → Findings: presents with fever +/- chills, facial pain and edema over the affected sinus, headaches, and purulent postnasal discharge → diagnosis: radiographs, CT scan (indicating **air-fluid level,** opacification of the sinus) → treatment: initially, the first few days may not require antibiotics due to viral sinusitis; if symptoms persist after 10 days, proceed to antibiotic therapy with **amoxicillin +/- clavulanate**.
- Chronic sinusitis => complication of acute sinusitis lasting for more than 4 weeks

- $\rightarrow$ Findings: similar to acute sinusitis $\rightarrow$ diagnosis: CT scan of the sinuses $\rightarrow$ treatment: Amoxicillin +/- clavulanate for 3 weeks $\rightarrow$ if there's no response, surgery may be beneficial.

- Acute otitis media => due to *S. pneumonia, H. influenza,* and *M. catarrhalis* $\rightarrow$ common in children and presents with nausea, vomiting, ear pain, and **bulging of the tympanic membrane which is difficult-to-see (light reflex)** $\rightarrow$ treatment: amoxicillin $\rightarrow$ complications: hearing loss, tympanic membrane perforation, mastoiditis, meningitis, venous thrombosis, cranial nerve VII and VIII palsies, and chronic otitis media $\rightarrow$ recommend tympanostomy tubes for patients with hearing loss or refractory to treatment.

- Otitis externa => mostly caused by *P. aeruginosa* $\rightarrow$ also known as the swimmer's ear; may be associated with trauma and foreign object $\rightarrow$ Findings: erythematous ear canal with pain and swelling, **foul smelling discharge, manipulation of auricle produces pain**, and hearing loss $\rightarrow$ treatment: Remove foreign object if present and topical antibiotics (neomycin or polymyxin B, ofloxacin).

- Ventilator-associated pneumonia (VAP) => common in the hospital-setting $\rightarrow$ caused by *S. aureus* (MRSA), *Legionella, Pseudomonas, Acinetobacter* $\rightarrow$ diagnosis: sputum culture $\rightarrow$ treatment: broad-spectrum antibiotic coverage until culture analysis becomes available.

- Tetanus prophylaxis => if immunization is **unknown** or patient has **< three doses**, give **tetanus vaccine + immunoglobulin** if the wound is dirty and prone to infection $\rightarrow$ however, clean wound should only get tetanus vaccine $\rightarrow$ also, if tetanus immunization history is known and patient has history of three or more doses, no immunoglobulin needed $\rightarrow$ if the wound is dirty, more than 24 hours since the wound injury, or > five years since the last booster, give tetanus vaccine $\rightarrow$ even if the wound is clean & the last booster given is > ten year, give tetanus booster $\rightarrow$ complications of tetanus include seizures + respiratory depression.

- Diverticulitis => inflammation of the diverticulum $\rightarrow$ Findings: fever, chills, nausea, vomiting, LLQ abdominal pain +/- diarrhea $\rightarrow$ diagnosis: clinical diagnosis or obtain a CT scan of the abdomen, CBC, blood cultures $\rightarrow$ treatment: Bowel rest, NPO, IVFs, and antibiotics (ciprofloxacin or metronidazole) $\rightarrow$ complication: diverticular abscess, sepsis, and death.

- Malaria prophylaxis => treat with mefloquine 1 week prior to travel $\rightarrow$ there are associated neuropsychiatric side effects with mefloquine.

- Traveler's diarrhea => treat symptomatic patients with TMP-SMX, fluoroquinolone (ciprofloxacin), or azithromycin.

- A prostitute with history of STDs and complaining of a rash, fever, arthralgia, and malaise, probably has syphilis!

- Fulminant hepatic failure => acute liver disease occurring in the absence of preexisting liver disease $\rightarrow$ leads to encephalopathy within 2 weeks of the onset of jaundice.

Chapter 9
Nephrology
<u>Acute Renal Failure (ARF)</u>

1. ARF usually occurs in the first few hours to days. Inability to produce urine is defined as **anuria** (< 100 cc), **oliguria** (100-400 cc), **non-oliguria** (400-1000 cc), and **polyuria** (> 1000 cc).
2. There are three categories: Prerenal, renal (intrinsic), and postrenal.
3. Findings: Dyspnea, fatigue, and presence of uremia (nausea, hyperpigmentation of skin, asterixis, and pericarditis).
4. Diagnosis: The lab generally shows the increase in creatinine and BUN, decrease in glomerular filtration rate, hyperkalemia, hypervolemia with symptoms of heart failure, and metabolic acidosis. Obtain electrolytes, BUN/creatinine, CBC, and urinalysis.
5. Treatment: Management includes monitoring electrolytes (calcium, phosphate, potassium); avoid offending/nephrotoxic drugs; watch contrast-study agents in renal disease; neutralize acidosis with sodium bicarbonate; and start dialysis when appropriate.

- **Prerenal: Most common is hypovolemia** (such as dehydration, hemorrhage) caused by **decreased renal perfusion**. Other causes are heart failure, liver failure, sepsis, and renovascular hypertension → **Findings:** tachycardia, weak/diminished pulses +/- heart failure symptoms → **diagnosis:** BUN/creatinine ratio > 20 → **treatment:** IVFs (in hypovolemia) and furosemide (in symptomatic heart failure).

- **Intrinsic (renal): Most common is acute tubular necrosis (ATN).** ATN is caused by toxins, ischemic damage, or medications such as NSAIDs, aminoglycosides, methicillin, and cyclosporine. **ATN** presents with **granular, muddy brown casts** and tubular epithelial cells. Other types of intrinsic are vascular, glomerular, or interstitial → **examples are: IV contrast** => remember to hydrate adequately before contrast study to prevent renal failure especially in diabetics; **glomerulonephritis** => in children after streptococcal infection and presents with **RBC casts**, edema, hematuria, and hypertension; **lupus erythematosus** => look for lupus symptoms + renal failure; **Goodpasture syndrome** => presents with dyspnea, hemoptysis, renal failure; **Wegener granulomatosis** => involves lung and kidney with sinonasal symptoms; **acute interstitial nephritis** => look for WBC casts and eosinophils in urinalysis; occurs 10-15 days after taking medication (NSAIDs).

- **Postrenal:** due to urinary outflow obstruction caused by benign prostatic hypertrophy (BPH) that leads to fluid overload from urinary retention → **Findings:** hesitancy, urgency, frequency, and anuria → **diagnosis:** assess postvoid residual with foley catheter, ultrasound, pyelography → **treatment:** catheterization and transurethral resection of the prostate (TURP).

Chronic Renal Failure

1. Chronic or prolonged damage to the kidney. Some of the causes are diabetes, polycystic kidney disease, and hypertension.
2. Findings: Similar to acute renal failure => dyspnea, fatigue, and presence of uremia (nausea, hyperpigmentation of skin, asterixis, and pericarditis). However, some patients may be asymptomatic.
3. Diagnosis: Look out for metabolic abnormalities => increase in creatinine and BUN, decrease in glomerular filtration rate, hyperkalemia, hypervolemia with symptoms of heart failure, metabolic acidosis, anemia (due to diminished erythropoietin), hypocalcemia & hyperphosphatemia (vitamin D production impairment), uremic pericarditis, bleeding (platelet dysfunction), and CNS toxicity (build-up of toxins). Obtain creatinine level; when > 1.4 mg/dL, it is considered renal failure.
4. Treatment: Dialysis, erythropoietin, vitamin D, calcium, and phosphate binders. Renal transplantation is the definitive treatment.

Urinary Tract Infection (UTI)

- Etiology: *E. coli* infection. Women are more susceptible to UTI than men because of their shorter urethra.
- Findings: Dysuria, urgency, frequency +/- suprapubic tenderness. Many patients are asymptomatic.
- Diagnosis: Urinalysis (shows WBCs, **nitrite**, leukocyte esterase, and bacteria) and **urine culture**.
- Treatment: TMP-SMX, ciprofloxacin for 7-10 days.

Nephrotic Syndrome

1. Daily excessive excretion of protein > 3.5 g/day.

2. Etiology (adults): Diabetes, drugs (penicillamine, gold), lupus, HIV; others are amyloidosis, minimal change (children), focal segmental glomerulosclerosis, membranous nephropathy, and membrano-proliferative nephropathy.
3. Findings: Edema +/- frothy urine.
4. Diagnosis: 24-hour urine protein, lipid panel, urinalysis (fat vacuoles in a Maltese cross pattern), BUN/creatinine, and electrolytes. Consider obtaining a renal biopsy. Remember to order tests for other causes such as ANA, RPR, beta HCG, fasting glucose, and liver enzymes.
5. Treatment: Treat underlying cause, statins for hyperlipidemia, control diabetes and use ACEIs for microalbuminuria. Heparin may be needed for hypercoagulable state.

- **Minimal change disease:** Occurs in children after an upper respiratory infection → Findings: edema +/- frothy urine → diagnosis: 24-hour urine protein, electron microscopy shows loss of podocyte foot processes → treatment: steroids.

- **Focal segmental glomerulosclerosis:** Idiopathic, HIV patient, IV drug abuser → diagnosis: urinalysis (hematuria) + renal biopsy (sclerosis in capillary tufts) → treatment: steroids.

- **Membranous nephropathy:** Immune-complex pathology → diagnosis: renal biopsy (**'spike and dome'** appearance, IgG & C3 deposit at the basement membrane) → treatment: Steroids → related to malaria, hepatitis B, syphilis, and gold.

- **Diabetic nephropathy:** Nodular glomerulosclerosis (Kimmelstiel-Wilson lesions) and diffuse hyalinization forms) → there's underlying history of diabetes → diagnosis: renal biopsy (thickened glomerular basement membrane) → treatment: manage diabetes effectively and initiate ACEIs for microalbuminuria.

- **Lupus nephritis:** Renal disease in lupus patients → diagnosis: urinalysis (proteinuria/RBCs), renal biopsy (subendothelial immune complex deposition) → treatment: steroids.

- **Renal amyloidosis:** Associated with multiple myeloma → diagnosis: Congo red stain, polarized light (apple-green birefringence), and abdominal fat biopsy → treatment: steroids, melphalan, and bone marrow transplant (for multiple myeloma).

- **Membrano-proliferative nephropathy** => Associated with hepatitis C, SLE, and cryoglobulinemia → diagnosis: C3 (decreased) and renal biopsy (**'tram-track' basement membrane**) → treatment: steroids → complication: slow progression to renal failure.

Nephrolithiasis

1. Kidney stones with risk factors: decreased fluid intake/dehydration, positive family history, gout, and chronic diarrhea.
2. Types of stones: **Calcium stones** (calcium oxalate/phosphate) can be seen in primary hyperparathyroidism and malignancy; observe for hypercalcemia. **Struvite (magnesium-ammonium-phosphate) stones** are related to ammonia-producing organisms (*Proteus*, *S. aureus*), staghorn calculi, radiopaque with alkaline urine. **Uric acid stones** are related to gout, hyperuricemia, leukemia (high purine turnover state, so give allopurinol before chemotherapy), and **alkalinize the urine with citrate**. **Cystine stones** are related to transport of amino acids, hexagonal crystals, and cystinuria; alkalinize the urine and treat with penicillamine. (**Most of the stones are radiodense except uric acid stone which is completely radiolucent**).
3. Findings: Severe, intermittent, colicky flank pain that may radiate to the groin area, +/- nausea and vomiting. Patients move around frequently to try to be comfortable; whereas in peritonitis, patients are lying down still and not moving. Observe for CVA tenderness.
4. Diagnosis: Urinalysis (to check hematuria and possible UTI), abdominal x-ray (**KUB** for radiopaque stones), **CT scan of the abdomen without contrast**, IV pyelogram (IVP; shows radiolucent stones). Also obtain calcium, BUN/creatinine, and CBC. Stones retrieved in urine should be analyzed.
5. Treatment: Lots of hydration, analgesics and stone (< 5 mm) may pass out through the urethra by itself. If not (> 3 cm), order shock-wave lithotripsy or percutaneous nephrolithotomy.

Pyelonephritis

1. Etiology: Caused by gram-negative bacteria (*E. coli, Klebsiella, Proteus*).
2. Findings: Patients are more ill-appearing; nausea, vomiting, fever, shaking chills, dysuria, **flank pain (CVA tenderness)**, with occasional diarrhea. Other possible symptoms are tachycardia and hypotension.
3. Diagnosis: Check for **bacteria in urine** with **leukocyte (WBCs) casts**, urine +/- blood culture.
4. Treatment: IV Fluoroquinolone or ceftriaxone during pregnancy.

Syndrome of Inappropriate Secretion of ADH (SIADH)

1. Hyponatremia that results from increased antidiuretic hormone (ADH).
2. Etiology: Head trauma, surgery, small cell cancer of the lung, brain abscess, meningitis, pneumonia, tuberculosis, postoperative after fluid administration or after painful episodes, and drugs (clofibrate, chlorpropamide, carbamazepine).
3. Findings: Asymptomatic is common; when serum sodium becomes < 120 mEq/L, patients usually become symptomatic, which involves the nervous system (seizures, mental status changes, confusion, lethargy, and coma).
4. Diagnosis: Serum sodium (< 135 mEq/L), plasma osmolality (< 270 mOsm/kg), urine osmolality (> 100 mOsm/kg). Patients usually become symptomatic with serum sodium < 120 mEq/L. (Normal serum sodium is 135-145 mEq/L).
5. Treatment: **Fluid (free-water) restriction**; if no response, administer **demeclocycline** (causes diabetes insipidus). Only symptomatic hyponatremia (**with seizures**) can be treated carefully with **hypertonic saline** (do **not use** normal saline here). Other times, normal saline is usually used.
6. Complication: **Central pontine myelinolysis** (brainstem damage due to rapid correction of hyponatremia).

Indications for Emergency Dialysis

1. Refractory hyperkalemia.
2. Refractory academia/acidosis.
3. Uremic pericarditis.
4. Volume overload.
5. Acute renal decompensation with mental status changes.
6. Serum creatinine greater than 10 mg/dL.
7. Serum BUN greater than 100 mg/dL.

Benign Prostatic Hypertrophy

1. Also known as Benign Prostatic Hyperplasia which leads to bladder outlet obstruction in men over the age of 40.

2. Findings: Urgency, frequency, and nocturia with feeling of incomplete emptying of the bladder.
3. Diagnosis: Urinalysis and PSA. PSA > 2.5 may be followed with transurethral biopsy.
4. Treatment: Terazosin (alpha blocker), finasteride (5-alpha reductase inhibitor), and transurethral resection of the prostate (TURP, for refractory cases). The side effects of TURP are retrograde ejaculation and hyponatremia.

Erectile Dysfunction

1. Patient is unable to have or maintain an erection and sometimes ejaculation.
2. Etiology: Psychological (**sudden with normal nocturnal penile tumescence** while patients with organic cause have abnormal nocturnal penile tumescence), organic (chronic; due to diabetes, atherosclerosis, stroke, multiple sclerosis, and seizures), and exogenous (clonidine, tricyclic antidepressants, alpha blockers, and anticholinergics).
3. Findings: normal/diminished peripheral pulses, skin atrophy, small testes, and hair loss.
4. Diagnosis: Glucose, prolactin, testosterone, and TSH.
5. Treatment: Sildenafil (PDE-5a inhibitor by inhibiting cGMP phosphodiesterase), testosterone, antidepressants, and anxiolytics. Vascular surgery may be beneficial. Remember to not combine sildenafil with nitrates or alpha blockers → causes hypotension, headaches, and flushing.

NEPHROLOGY 1-LINER JUNKY CASES

- **Hyponatremia** => serum sodium < 135 mEq/L → asymptomatic is common; when serum sodium becomes < 120 mEq/L, patients usually become symptomatic, which involves the nervous system (seizures, mental status changes, confusion, lethargy, and coma).
- **Hypernatremia** => serum sodium > 147 mEq/L → patients have symptoms as in hyponatremia which includes seizures, mental status changes, confusion, lethargy, and coma.
- **Hypocalcemia** => symptoms of tetany, carpal spasm, dementia, depression, convulsions, and encephalopathy → order ECG (shows **prolonged QT interval**).
- **Hypercalcemia** => asymptomatic is common → due to hyperparathyroidism, vitamin D toxicity, sacordosis, thiazide, cancer, and familial hypocalciuric hypercalcemia → hypercalcemia presents with '**bones, stones, groans,** and **psychiatric overtones**' → order ECG (shows **short QT interval**). In a patient who is hypercalcemic and presenting with symptoms (nausea, vomiting, tachycardia), initiate **IV hydration**. Do not use bisphosphonate because this is used for maintenance of chronic hypercalcemia and not acute hypercalcemia; besides bisphosphonate takes about 2 weeks to work.
- **Hypokalemia** => serum potassium < 3.5 mEq/L → presents with muscular cramps or weakness, ileus, hyporeflexia, and flaccid paralysis → order ECG (shows **T-wave flattening, U waves** → watch in patients on diuretics or in anorexia.
- **Hyperkalemia** => serum potassium > 5 mEq/L → presents mainly with **weakness/paralysis** → order ECG (shows **tall, peaked T waves** and **widening of QRS complex**) → watch in renal failure patients, rhabdomyolysis, drugs (NSAIDs, ACEIs), and Addison disease (adrenal insufficiency) → treatment: calcium gluconate, then sodium bicarbonate +/- glucose and insulin.
- **Goodpasture syndrome** => Findings: dyspnea, hemoptysis, renal failure → diagnosis: renal biopsy shows linear immunofluorescence pattern, antiglomerular basement membrane antibodies → treatment: steroids +/- cyclophosphamide.
- **Wegener granulomatosis** => involves lung and kidney → Findings: hemoptysis, sinonasal symptoms (sinusitis, **bleeding of the nose**, and **nasal perforation**) → diagnosis: **positive antineutrophilic cytoplasmic antibody (ANCA)** titer → treatment: cyclophosphamide.
- **Glomerulonephritis** => in children after streptococcal infection → Findings: edema, hematuria, and hypertension → diagnosis: **RBC casts**, urinalysis with hematuria → treatment: supportively.
- **NSAIDs** can cause papillary necrosis → it also causes afferent arteriolar vasoconstriction.
- **Renal Tubular Acidosis (RTA)** => decrease in tubular hydrogen secretion or bicarbonate reabsorption that leads to non-anion gap metabolic acidosis.

- Rhabdomyolysis => caused by strenuous exercise → Findings: nausea, muscle pain → diagnosis: increased creatine phosphokinase (CPK) or creatine kinase (CK) and myoglobinuria → treatment: hydration and diuretics.
- Hematuria without other lab abnormality should be rechecked → therefore, repeat urinalysis → isolated hematuria is seen in strenuous exercise.
- **Persistent hematuria** should be worked up using renal ultrasound, IVP, cystoscopy, and renal angiogram.
- Remember, sometimes foods, drugs, or dyes can falsely cause hematuria.
- Pyelonephritis lasting more than 48 hours may be due to renal abscess → order CT scan; if positive, order surgical drainage.
- Consider treating asymptomatic pregnant patients with UTIs to prevent pyelonephritis → treatment: amoxicillin.
- Nephritic syndrome => caused by poststreptococcal glomerulonephritis → Findings: oliguria + increased BUN/creatinine + hematuria + hypertension → diagnosis: urinalysis (RBC casts), which indicates glomerulonephritis.
- Oxytocin given during labor → and several hours later, there's seizure + hyponatremia → treatment: stop oxytocin.
- Polycystic kidney disease patients are at risk of subarachnoid hemorrhage and diverticular disease.
- IgA nephropathy => URIs + hematuria + presents with normal complement levels.
- Poststreptococcal glomerulonephritis => usually presents 10-14 days after an acute streptococcal pharyngitis.

Chapter 10
Pediatrics

Immunization Vaccines

Vaccine	When to Administer
Hepatitis B	3 doses: Administered initially at birth (0), 1-4, and 6-18 months of age
Diphtheria, tetanus, pertussis (DTaP)	5 doses: Administered at 2, 4, 6, 15-18 months; and 4-6 years of age, then every 10 years
Polio (IPV)	4 doses: Administered at 2, 4, 6 months, 4-6 years of age
H. influenzae type b (Hib)	4 doses: Administered at 2, 4, 6 months, 12-15 months of age
Measles, mumps, rubella (MMR)	2 doses: Administered at 12-15 months, 4-6 years of age
Varicella	1 dose: Administered at 12-18 months of age
Pneumococcal vaccine (conjugate)	4 doses: Administered at 2, 4, 6, 12-15 months of age
Rotavirus	3 doses: Administered at 2, 4, 6 months of age
Influenza	Administered after 6 months of age, then yearly

Preventive Health and Screening in Pediatrics

*****Routinely, assessing the overall developmental progress and well-being of a child after birth is vital. The following should be considered:

1. **Metabolic/congenital diseases** => screening for congenital hypothyroidism and phenylketonuria within the first month of life are part of all states screening. Other testing varies from state to state.

2. Growth (height, weight, circumference of the head) and developmental milestones should be measured at least every 6 months until the age of three for head circumference, and until adulthood for the height and weight.

3. **Anemia** => routine screening is controversial; screening is generally recommended for children at risk of iron deficiency (poor iron intake, prematurity, and cow milk intake before the age of 1). Iron supplements may be needed.

4. **Lead** => routine screening is controversial; screening is recommended for high-risk children (such as those living in old buildings). Measure lead levels (normal is < 10 ug/dL) and remove the child from the building.

5. **Anticipatory guidance** => the goal is to take necessary precautions to try to prevent disasters. Remember, car accidents (**use car seats**, placed in rear of car, without airbag, and rear-facing until 1 year of age), put the baby to sleep supine (prevents SIDS), watch for small objects (can cause aspiration), cleaning chemicals (can cause burns), and supervise baths (avoid drowning). Others are nutrition (avoid cow milk before the age of 1 (causes iron deficiency anemia) and start solid foods at 6 months of age.

6. **Vision and hearing** => start hearing and vision screening at birth, age of three, then every two years until adolescent.

7. **Vitamin D** => recommended for children with minimal sun exposure, inadequate maternal intake, and prolonged breastfeeding beyond 6 months of age.

8. **Fluoride** => supplementation is usually needed in underserved/rural areas.

9. **Tuberculosis (TB)** => screen annually only in high-risk children (such as HIV infection) with PPD skin test.

10. **STD screening** => controversial; but where needed, may start screening at 11 years of age, which may also include a urinalysis.

Neonatal Infections-T.O.R.C.H.S
Toxoplasmosis

1. Etiology: Exposure to cat feces during pregnancy, raw or undercooked meat.
2. Findings: Seizures, chorioretinitis, intracranial calcifications, and hydrocephalus.
3. Diagnosis: CT scan of the head (intracranial calcifications and ring-enhancing lesions).
4. Treatment: Pyrimethamine and sulfadiazine.

Non-T.OR.C.H.S Infections

1. Infections include HIV, varicella, tuberculosis, parvovirus, *Listeria*, and fungal.
2. Findings: Depends on the underlying infection/disease.
3. Diagnosis: Initially, CBC, electrolytes, urinalysis, PPD skin test.
4. Treatment: Depends on the underlying infection/disease.

Rubella (German Measles)

1. Findings: Low-grade fever, painful and swelling of the **suboccipital and postauricular nodes**.
2. Diagnosis: Screen and **immunize women** of reproductive age **prior to pregnancy**. Check maternal rubella antibody during the first prenatal visit.
3. Treatment: Supportively.
4. Complications: **Otitis media** and **encephalitis**. Also evaluate neonates for **cardiovascular defects** (patent ductus and ventricular septal defect), **deafness**, microphthalmia, and cataracts.

Cytomegalovirus (CMV)

1. Findings: Deafness, petechial rash, microphthalmia, chorioretinitis, periventricular/intracranial calcifications, and microcephaly.
2. Diagnosis: CT scan of the head.
3. Treatment: Ganciclovir.

Herpes

1. Etiology: History of maternal genital herpes.
2. Findings: Skin vesicular lesions (may appear on the eyes, mouth, and face).
3. Diagnosis: Tzanck smears (positive for lesions).
4. Treatment: Acyclovir.

Syphilis

1. Findings: Maculopapular skin rash, **lymphadenopathy**, rhinitis, **saber shins**, **Hutchinson teeth**, and interstitial keratitis.
2. Diagnosis: VDRL

3. Treatment: IM penicillin.

Neonatal Respiratory Distress

1. Etiology: **Meconium aspiration syndrome** (inhalation of meconium), **transient tachypnea of the newborn** (fluid in fetal lung), **respiratory distress syndrome** or **hyaline membrance disease** (surfactant deficiency), and **congenital diaphragmatic hernia** (abdominal contents in chest cavity leading to pulmonary hypoplasia; shows as cystic mass in chest similar to bowel loops).
2. Findings: Dyspnea/respiratory distress are common in all types.
3. Diagnosis: Obtain chest x-ray.
4. Treatment: **Nasopharyngeal suctioning** (for meconium aspiration syndrome); **steroids and surfactant** (for respiratory distress syndrome); **oxygen** (for transient tachypnea of the newborn); **intubation, ventilatory support,** and **surgery** (for congenital diaphragmatic hernia).

Neonatal Sepsis

1. Risk factors: Positive maternal group B streptoccal (GBS) infection (screened at 36 weeks gestation), maternal fever, prolonged rupture of the membranes > 18 hours, chorioamnionitis, and preterm labor.
2. Etiology: *E. coli*, group B streptococcal infection, and *Listeria monocytogenes*.
3. Findings: Fever, respiratory distress, and poor feeding.
4. Diagnosis: Blood and urine cultures, urinalysis, CBC, chest x-ray, and CSF culture by lumbar puncture.
5. Treatment: **Ampicillin + gentamicin** or ampicillin + third-generation cephalosporin for *Listeria*. If UTI is the cause of sepsis, obtain VCUG and renal ultrasound to check for vesicoureteral reflux and hydronephrosis respectively. **GBS is treated** prophylactically with **penicillin** during labor and upon delivery to prevent neonatal sepsis.

Neonatal Jaundice
Physiologic Jaundice

1. Unconjugated/indirect hyperbilirubinemia in neonates that **starts in the first two days (day 1-2) of life** and **peaks by day 5**. It returns to normal by day 14.
2. Findings: There is jaundice from the head to the eyes and body, poor feeding,

seizures, and flaccidity.

3. Diagnosis: Bilirubin levels (increased 10-15 mg/dl) and peripheral blood smear to distinguish between conjugated and unconjugated hyperbilirubinemia.
4. Treatment: **UV phototherapy** and exchange transfusion if severe.
5. Complications: Encephalopathy (**kernicterus**) from deposit of bilirubin into the basal ganglia.

Breast Milk Jaundice

1. Usually occurs **after 14 days of life** → infants are breastfed.
2. Diagnosis: Diagnosis of exclusion; bilirubin levels (increased, 10-20 mg/dl).
3. Treatment: Temporarily, stop breastfeeding until jaundice resolves. However, may require phototherapy if no resolution.

Pathologic Jaundice

1. Conjugated/direct hyperbilirubinemia as a result of underlying disorder.
2. Etiology: Biliary atresia (**most common**), cystic fibrosis, hypothyroidism, hemolysis secondary to Rh incompatibility, metabolic (Criggler-Najjar disease, Gilbert disease), alpha1-antitrypsin deficiency, neonatal hepatitis, and medications (sulfa drugs).
3. Findings: Jaundice, poor feeding, seizures, high-pitched cry, and splenomegaly.
4. Diagnosis: CBC (check for anemia), Coomb's test (differentiates immune- vs non-immune diseases), and peripheral smear (check for hemolysis).
5. Treatment: Phototherapy and exchange transfusion.

Pediatrics Cardiology
Ventricular Septal Defect (VSD)

1. VSD is the **most common** congenital heart defect → defect is a hole in the ventricular septum.
2. Findings: Remember small defects may be asymptomatic. Patients with symptoms have **vibratory holosystolic or pansystolic murmur at left lower sternum border**, failure to thrive, exercise or feeding intolerance. Watch for symptoms of heart failure (dyspnea, peripheral edema) if the defect is large.

3. Diagnosis: **ECG** (indicating hypertrophies of the left and right ventricles) and echocardiography.
4. Treatment: **Furosemide** (for heart failure), **schedule follow-up visits for small VSDs** annually (they may resolve spontaneously), and **surgery** for larger defects.
5. Complications: VSDs that are left untreated may result in triad of pulmonary hypertension, right ventricular hypertrophy (RVH), and reversal of right-to-left shunt (known as **Eisenmenger's syndrome**).

Atrial Septal Defect (ASD)

1. Congenital heart defect from a hole in the atrial septum.
2. Findings: The child may be asymptomatic until adulthood; **fixed split S2 and palpitations, systolic ejection murmur at the left upper sternal border.**
3. Diagnosis: ECG (left axis deviation), chest x-ray (increased pulmonary markings), and echocardiography.
4. Treatment: **Furosemide** (for heart failure), **schedule follow-up visits for small ASDs** annually, and **surgery** for large defects.
5. Complication: Eisenmenger's syndrome.

Patent Ductus Arteriosus (PDA)

1. The ductus arteriosus failed to close in the first day of life → resulting to a left-to-right shunt.
2. Risk factors: Prematurity, congenital rubella infection, and high altitude.
3. Findings: Look out for **continuous machinery murmur** in the left upper sternal border, **wide pulse pressure**, dyspnea +/- symptoms of heart failure.
4. Diagnosis: Echocardiography (shows shunt from left atrium to right atrium).
5. Treatment: Indomethacin (closes PDA), surgery (if medication fails).
6. If there is transposition of great arteries that is dependent on PDA, keep it **open** with prostaglandin E1.

Tetralogy of Fallot (TOF)

1. TOF is the **most common cyanotic congenital heart defect**.
2. It consists of pulmonary stenosis (right ventricle outflow obstruction), right ventricle hypertrophy, overriding aorta, and ventricular septal defect.

3. Findings: **Squatting after exertion** such as playing or running (**"tet spells"**), cyanosis, **systolic ejection murmur** at the left sternal border, and a single S2 heart sound.
4. Diagnosis: Chest x-ray (shows boot-shaped heart) and echocardiography (**definitive test**).
5. Treatment: Prostaglandin E1 helps to resolve cyanosis, oxygen, continue squatting as needed, IVFs, morphine, and surgical repair.

Coarctation of the Aorta

1. Etiology: Due to the narrowing of the lumen of the aorta and resulting in decreased blood flow below the obstruction and increased flow above the obstruction.
2. Risk factor: Turner syndrome. It is associated with **bicuspid aortic valve**.
3. Findings: **Dyspnea on exertion**, **upper extremities hypertension** and lower extremities hypotension/lower blood pressures, **decreased femoral** and **distal lower extremity pulses** +/- syncope.
4. Diagnosis: Chest x-ray (rib notching) and echocardiography/catheterization.
5. Treatment: Surgical repair/balloon angioplasty.
6. Remember to give dental prophylaxis with amoxicillin.

Transposition of the Great Arteries

1. Etiology: The defect lies with the aorta forming from the right ventricle, and the pulmonary artery is forming from the left ventricle → leading to severe cyanosis.
2. Findings: **Severe cyanosis** and a **single S2 heart sound**.
3. Diagnosis: Chest x-ray (shows **egg-on-a-string**) and echocardiography (**definitive test**).
4. Treatment: Prostaglandin (to open PDA) and surgical repair.

Pediatrics Pulmonology
Croup (Acute Laryngotracheobronchitis)

1. Inflammatory disease of the larynx or subglottic that usually occurs in the fall or winter and affects patients 1-2 years of age.
2. Etiology: Due to parainfluenza virus (**mostly,** 50-70%) or influenza.
3. Findings: Starts with viral/upper respiratory infection symptoms of low-grade fever, cough, rhinorrhea that progresses to hoarseness, **barking cough**, and inspiratory stridor.
4. Diagnosis: Consider clinical findings; AP lateral x-ray of the neck (shows **'steeple sign'** indicating narrowing of the subglottic due to edema).
5. Treatment: Humidified oxygen with mist therapy, aerosolized racemic epinephrine, and corticosteroids (dexamethasone).

Epiglottitis

1. Infection of the epiglottis leading to severe airway obstruction that usually affects patients between 2-7 years of age.
2. Etiology: *H. influenza* type b (**mostly**), *S. pneumonia,* and *S. aureus.*
3. Findings: Sudden-onset of high fever, **drooling**, toxic appearance with inspiratory retractions/respiratory distress, and +/- cyanosis.
4. Diagnosis: Based on clinical findings; to avoid worsening airway obstruction, **do not examine the throat until the patient is in the operating room, and the specialist is prepared to establish the airway**. However, lateral neck x-ray (shows "**thumbprint**" **sign** indicating swollen epiglottis).
5. Treatment: **Endotracheal intubation** or tracheostomy (once in the OR, by the anesthesiologist) and IV antibiotics (third-generation cephalosporin).

Respiratory Syncytial Virus (RSV)

1. Also known as bronchiolitis that affects children < 18 months of age in the fall or winter.
2. Etiology: Mostly respiratory syncytial virus (RSV); other causes are *parainfluenza* and *influenza.*
3. Findings: Rapid inspirations, **expiratory wheezing**, and intercoastal retractions.
4. Diagnosis: PCR for RSV using nasopharyngeal swap and chest x-ray (shows **diffuse hyperinflation**, flattened diaphragms).
5. Treatment: Supportively with **humidified oxygen, IVFs, saline nasal drops**, and **albuterol**. Ribavarin may be required for severe cases and endotracheal intubation if there is respiratory arrest.

Pertussis

1. Known as the contagious "whooping cough."
2. Etiology: *Bordetella pertussis*.
3. Findings: Severe paroxysmal coughing with a loud whooping inspiratory noise.
4. Diagnosis: PCR for *B. pertussis* using nasopharyngeal swap.
5. Treatment: Azithromycin.
6. Patients with diphtheria, caused by *Corynebacterium diphtheria*, presents with **grayish pseudomembranes** on uvula, tonsils, and pharynx. Combination of pertussis and diphtheria are usually present in patients without immunizations.

Pediatrics Gastroenterology
Intussusception

1. Twisting of the bowel segment → intussusception is the **most common cause of obstruction** in the first two years of life.
2. Findings: **Currant-jelly stools**, vomiting, **palpable sausage-like mass**, with paroxysmal abdominal pain.
3. Diagnosis & Treatment: Air-contrast enema or barium enema (diagnostic and therapeutic).
4. Complication: Gut necrosis and death.

Pyloric Stenosis

1. Etiology: Due to the hypertrophy of the pylorus that results in gastric obstruction in mostly male infants in the first three weeks of life.
2. Findings: **Palpable olive-shaped mass** in the epigastrium with visible peristaltic waves; **non-bilious projectile** vomiting.
3. Diagnosis: **Abdominal ultrasound** (shows hypertrophied pylorus), electrolytes (shows **hypochloremic, hypokalemic metabolic alkalosis** suggesting underlying vomiting), and barium enema (shows "**string sign**", narrowing of the pylorus).
4. Treatment: Hydration, replacement of electrolytes as needed, and surgery (pyloromyotomy).

Malrotation or Volvulus

1. Etiology: Abnormal rotation of the stomach and incomplete fixation to the posterior of the abdominal wall.
2. Findings: Can occur from the first three weeks of life to two years of age; sudden onset of abdominal pain and distention, **bilious vomiting**, obstruction, peritonitis, +/- rectal bleeding.
3. Diagnosis: Upper GI series, barium enema (shows **mobile** cecum), and contrast studies (show "bird's beak" in small bowel).
4. Treatment: Surgery.
5. Complication: Gut necrosis.

Necrotizing Enterocolitis

1. Necrosis of the intestine in watershed distributions.
2. Risk factors: Premature infants and congenital heart defects.
3. Findings: Fever, poor feeding, air in bowel wall/abdominal distention, rectal bleeding, and hypotension or shock.
4. Diagnosis: Abdominal x-ray (shows **pneumatosis intestinalis** = air in the intestine).
5. Treatment: NPO, orogastric tube, IVFs, antibiotics, and surgery (if bowel is necrotic).

Meckel's Diverticulum

1. Outpouching of the distal ileum from the **remnant of the omphalomesenteric duct** → contains ectopic (pancreatic/gastric) mucosa. It is the **most common GI tract abnormality**.
2. It consists of the 'rule of 2's': 2 feet proximal to the ileocecal valve, 2% of population affected, 2 inches long, 2 cm in diameter, and presents by age 2.
3. Findings: **Painless rectal bleeding**; GI bleeding, gastric ulceration, obstruction, or volvulus may also be present.
4. Diagnosis: Meckel's scan (to detect bleeding) or tissue biopsy (definitive test).
5. Treatment: IVFs, blood transfusion if needed, and surgery.

Kawasaki Disease

1. Also known as mucocutaneous lymph node syndrome affecting children < 5

years of age usually among Asians.

2. Findings: **Fever > 5 days, bilateral conjunctivitis**, changes in the tongue ('**strawberry tongue**', lips, and oral mucosa, swelling of the hands and feet, rash on the trunk, and cervical lymphadenopathy.
3. Diagnosis: Clinical diagnosis → may check ESR (increased).
4. Treatment: Aspirin and IV immune globulin. Follow-up with echocardiography to evaluate heart complications.
5. Complications: **Coronary artery aneurysms, heart failure,** and myocardial infarction.

Pediatrics Oncology
Wilms' Tumor

1. Most common **renal tumor** in children between 1-4 years of age.
2. Etiology: **Kidney** (embryonal origin) → risk factors include positive family history, neurofibromatosis, and other congenital anomalies such as Denys Drash syndrome and WAGR syndrome).
3. Findings: **Abdominal flank mass**, abdominal distention, hematuria, and hypertension.
4. Diagnosis: Abdominal ultrasound or **CT scan** of the abdomen (**preferred**), chest x-ray, chest CT scan, CBC, electrolytes, BUN/creatinine, liver enzymes, tissue biopy (**confirms**).
5. Treatment: **Transabdominal nephrectomy**, then chemotherapy (vincristine, dactinomycin) +/- flank irradiation with overall good prognosis depending on the severity/pathology of the tumor.

Neuroblastoma

1. Etiology: **Adrenal gland** (neural crest cell origin) tumor → can occur in children < 6 months of age up to 5 years of age. It is the **most common tumor** in **infants** and **of the adrenal gland**.
2. Risk factors: Neurofibromatosis, pheochromocytoma, Hirschsprung's disease, and tuberous sclerosis.
3. Findings: Abdominal/flank mass, abdominal distention, dyspnea, fatigue, weight loss, and +/- neurological symptoms.
4. Diagnosis: 24-hour urinary catecholamines (shows **increased VMA** and **HVA**), CT scan of the abdomen, chest x-ray, bone scan, CBC, electrolytes, BUN/creatinine, PT, PTT, and liver enzymes.
5. Treatment: Surgical excision and chemotherapy (cyclophosphamide, doxorubicin) +/- radiation.

PEDIATRICS 1-LINER JUNKY CASES

- Failure to thrive => inability for a child to grow in height or gain weight due to genetic disorder, growth hormone deficiency, or inadequate nutrition → a concern should rise when a previously growing child is experiencing slow growth → obtain nutrition and family history, and perform a complete physical examination → diagnosis: start with CBC, chemistry, and urinalysis → treatment: identify & treat the underlying cause, calorie count, nutritional supplementation, and hospital admission if necessary.

- Precocious puberty => idiopathic → may also be due to **McCune-Albright syndrome** that presents with café-au-lait spots, fibrous dysplasia, estrogen-secreting ovarian tumors → precocious puberty is also related to **congenital hyperplasia (CAH)** which is defined as ambigious genitalia, 21-hydroxylase deficiency, increased 17-hydroxyprogesterone, hypotension, and hyperkalemia; treat CAH with steroids and IVFs.

- **Child abuse** => Usually there is history given that does not match with the physical findings → considered as emotional, physical, sexual, and neglect → Findings: failure to thrive, injuries in various stages of healing, cigarette burns, retinal hemorrhage, bone fractures, and genital trauma with signs of STDs → diagnosis: ophthalmology exam, skeletal survey, and CT scan of the head → treatment: treat first, then report any suspected abuse or non-accidental trauma to Child Protective Services or social services; hospitalization may be needed to ensure the safety of the child.

- Omphalocele => membrane-covered and herniation of multiple abdominal organs which are midline → look for other congenital anomalies.

- Gastroschisis => intestinal organs are exposed, and there is no membrane/hernia sac.

- Hirschsprung's disease => infant is unable to pass meconium; absence of ganglion cells in the colon that leads to narrowing of the aganglionic segment, then dilation of proximal part of the colon → Findings: vomiting, abdominal distention, obstipation → diagnosis: **rectal biopsy** for ganglion cells → treatment: **staged surgery with initial diverting colostomy** and later with resection after 6 months of age.

- Tracheoesophageal fistula => esophagus with blind pouch proximally and a fistula between the distal esophagus and trachea → Findings: neonate presents with **excessive oral secretions**, choking, coughing, cyanosis with feedings, admonial distention, and respiratory distress → diagnosis: **nasogastric tube** (**can't pass through to the stomach**) and x-ray → treatment: surgery.

- Biliary atresia => Conjugated hyperbilirubinemia → Findings: Bilious vomiting, abdominal distention, clay-colored stools, and polyhydramnios → diagnosis: abdominal x-ray → treatment: surgery.

- Febrile seizures => seizures that are caused by fever and occur between 9 months and 5 years of age → the types are 1) **simple:** (short generalized seizure lasting 15 minutes without residual focal neurological deficit); treat by identifying source of fever → 2) **complex:** (long focal seizure lasting longer than 15 minutes **with some focal neurological deficit**; treat with acetaminophen and order CBC, blood cultures, electrolytes, urinalysis, EEG, MRI, lumbar puncture.

- Absence seizures => patients have brief staring episodes with rapid blinks of the eyelids that last 5-15 seconds → diagnosis: EEG shows generalized, 3-Hz spike and wave pattern → treatment: Ethosuximide.

- Infantile spasms => associated with **tuberous sclerosis** (hypopigmented skin macules/flesh colored papules on nasolabial fold, facial angiofibromas, seizures, mental retardation, CNS hamartoma, cardiac rhabdomyomas, and renal angiomyolipomas) → Findings: presents as "**jackknife**" spasms and developmental regression diagnosis: EEG shows **hypsarrhythmia** → treatment: ACTH.

- Trisomy 21 => (Down syndrome) → is the most common cause of mental retardation → Findings: hypotonia, transverse palmar crease, brachycephalic head, congenital heart defects, and GI (duodenal) atresia → diagnosis: karyotype, TFTs, and echocardiogram → associated with **leukemia** and **Alzheimer disease**.

- Trisomy 18 => (Edward syndrome) → mental retardation, microcephaly, clenched fist or overlapping third and fourth fingers, mental retardation, **rocker-bottom feet**, low-set ears → diagnosis: karyotype.

- Trisomy 13 => (Patau syndrome) → mental retardation, seizures, microphthalmia, **cleft lip or palate**, holoprosencephaly, and deafness → diagnosis: karyotype with FISH analysis.

- Turner syndrome => (45 XO) → short-stature, webbed neck, wide-spaced nipples, mental retardation, gonadal dysgenesis, congenital lymphedema, infertility, and coarctation of the aorta → diagnosis: karyotype.

- Carvenous hemangioma => in the first few days of life, the tumor becomes larger → **resolves spontaneously** → treat by **observing** and **follow-up.**

- Choanal atresia => occurs in the first week of life → presents as **inability to pass**

NGT through nose, cyanosis with feeding, infant feels relieved by crying.

- Henoch-Schonlein purpura => associated with IgA-mediated immune vasculitis → presents with abdominal pain + GI bleed + arthritis + hematuria + **rash on lower extremities and buttocks** + recent history of URI/GI infection → treatment: supportively (self-limiting disease) → most common cause of morbidity and mortality is **renal failure** in some patients.

- Infant botulism => due to **ingestion of honey or canned foods** that leads to sudden onset of muscle paralysis → diagnosis: *Clostridium botulinum* toxin → treatment: supportively with admission, close observation +/- intubation for respiratory muscle paralysis → child is expected to recover within a week.

- X-linked (Bruton's agammaglobulinemia) => is X-linked recessive disorder that usually presents in boys after 6 months of age, but may present earlier → there is **low or absent of B cells** → Findings: recurrent URIs → risk of pseudomonal infection → diagnosis: quantitative Ig levels.

- IgA deficiency => **most common immunodeficiency disorder** → usually asymptomatic, but may present with recurrent URIs and GI infections → diagnosis: low IgA → remember patients who have anaphylaxis reaction after immunoglobulin therapy may have IgA deficiency.

- Common variable immunodeficiency (CVID) => low levels of Igs between 20-30 years of age → there is risk of lymphoma and autoimmune disease.

- DiGeorge syndrome (Thymic aplasia) => patients do not have a thymus; therefore, unable to generate T cells → presents with tetany (hypocalcemia) → treatment: thymus transplant.

- Ataxia-telangiectasia => patient presents with ataxia + bilateral telangiectasis of the conjunctiva + history of URIs → associated with thymic hypoplasia.

- Severe combined immunodeficiency (SCID) => X-linked or **autosomal recessive** disorder (most common, due to adenosine deaminase deficiency) → due to **severe lack of B and T cells**, there is severe and recurrent bacterial and **fungal** infections → treatment: BMT.

- Wiskott-Aldrich syndrome => X-linked recessive disorder with impairment in the formation of antibodies to the polysaccharide capsular antigens → presents with **eczema, recurrent infections,** and **thrombocytopenia** → diagnosis: increased (IgE, IgA) and decreased IgM → treatment: IVIG and antibiotics.

- Chronic granulomatous disease (CGD) => X-linked or autosomal recessive disorder → due to deficient superoxide reduction by PMNs and macrophages → diagnosis: **deficient nitroblue tetrazolium dye reduction** by granulocyte →

treatment: TMP-SMX, antibiotics, and interferon.

- Chediak-Higashi syndrome => autosomal recessive disorder that is due to defect in neutrophil chemotaxis/microtubule polymerization → presents with recurrent skin and URIs, **oculocutaneous albinism**, neutropenia, and neuropathy → diagnosis: peripheral blood smear (**giant cytoplasmic granules in neutrophils**) → treatment: antibiotics, corticosteroids, and splenectomy.

- Terminal complement deficiency (C5-C9) => presents with recurrent infections by *Nisseria* spp. including gonococcal and meningococcal → diagnosis: total hemolytic complement, CH 50 → treatment: antibiotics and meningococcal vaccine.

- Measles (rubeola) => presents with high fever, malaise, cough, coryza, rhinitis, conjunctivitis, photophobia → after 72 hours of symptoms, there is white tiny spots on buccal mucosa (**koplik spots**), then maculopapular rash from head to trunk fashion → treatment: **supportively** → complication: otitis media, pneumonia, encephalitis (subacute sclerosing panencephalitis), pericarditis, and hepatitis → measles is associated with **vitamin A** deficiency.

- Roseola infantum (exanthema subitum) => due to **human herpesvirus type 6** → high-fever progresses > 40°C for 4 days without a cause → macular or maculopapular rash appears on the trunk and temperature returns to normal.

- Erythema infectiosum (fifth disease) => due to **parvovirus B19** → presents with low-grade fever, malaise, and erythema over the cheeks "**slapped-cheek**" rash → within 24-hour, maculopapular rash appears on the arms, legs, and trunk.

- Infectious mononucleosis => due to infection of EBV → presents with fever, pharyngitis/sore throat, generalized lymphadenopathy, **splenomegaly**, hepatomegaly, thrombocytopenia, → diagnosis: **atypical lymphocytes** with lymphocytosis on **peripheral blood smear**, Monospot test or EBV nuclear antigen → associated with **nasopharyngeal carcinoma** and **Burkitt lymphoma** → remember, patient should **avoid contact sports** to prevent splenic rupture.

- Scarlet fever => due to untreated streptococcal pharyngitis with presence of **erythrogenic toxin** → then, there is the appearance of sandpaper-like rash on the abdomen and trunk area with **circumoral pallor** + strawberry tongue; later, the fever resolves and the rash desquamates → treatment: prophylaxis with penicillin.

- Slipped capital femoral epiphysis => common in overweight males in ages 9-13 years old → presents with limp, knee and groin pain → diagnosis: AP pelvis x-ray (may be initially normal) → treatment: surgical pinning.

- Legg-Calve-Perthes disease => occurs mostly in short males with delayed bone age → presents with limp, knee and groin pain → treatment: **orthoses**.

- Congenital hip dysplasia => occurs at birth in first-born females during breech delivery → presents with Barlow's and Ortolani's signs → treatment: **harness** (orthopedic referral).

- Leukocoria => many WBCs in the anterior chamber → associated with retinoblastoma → diagnosis: obtain **CT scan of the orbits** to rule out retinoblastoma, ophthalmology eye exam, and x-ray of the globe for calcification.

- Prader-Willi syndrome => associated with the deletion of chromosome 15 → presents with hypoglycemia, hypotonia shortly after birth, poor feedings, and growth restriction → patients are **obese** and **develop sleep apnea**.

- Cystic fibrosis => due to mutation of the CF transmembrane regulator (CFTR) gene on chromosome 7 → presents with failure to thrive, malabsorption, history of URIs/pneumonia → diagnosis: sweat chloride test.

- Cryptorchidism => undescended testis in children should be referred to an urologist → treatment: exploratory laparotomy with orchioplexy.

- Testicular torsion => erythematous, swollen, tender testicle/scrotum with an **absent cremasteric reflex** → treatment: surgical evaluation.

- Meconium ileus => common in newborns with abdominal distention, vomiting, and failure to pass meconium in the first 48 hours of life → diagnosis: abdominal x-ray shows dilated loops of small bowel with air-fluid levels and a collection of "ground glass" appearance in the lower abdomen → associated with **cystic fibrosis**.

- Shaken baby syndrome => associated with subdural hematomas + retinal hemorrhages.

- The most common **abdominal mass** in a **newborn** => hydronephrosis.

- Viral conjunctivitis => associated with preauricular adenopathy.

- Rheumatic fever => there is history of streptococcal pharyngitis → other symptoms are polyathralgias, erythema marginatum, subcutaneous nodules, chorea, and carditis.

Chapter 11
Obstetrics
Prenatal Care

1. During the **first prenatal visit**, initial lab (**usually done during week 8-12**) should include pap smear, gonorrhea and chlamydia cultures, CBC, urinalysis, hepatitis B surface antigen, HIV, RPR, HSV type II, rubella antibody titer, blood type, Rh antibody, and **transvaginal** (can detect fetus as early as 5 weeks) or transabdominal ultrasound for gestational age. Also screen for diabetes (if obese or positive family history), sickle cell, and toxoplasmosis in high-risk patients. **Chronic villus sampling** (**CVS**) is done with the use of an ultrasound and aspiration of chorionic villus tissue during **week 10-12** to evaluate any genetic disease before an amniocentesis can be done. CVS causes **distal limb defects**.

2. **By week 15-20:** Obtain the **triple-marker screen test** or the quadruple test quad screen. Also obtain **screening ultrasound** for fetal anatomy, amniotic fluid, and placental location. The triple-marker screen consists of **maternal serum AFP**, estriol, and beta HCG. An **increased AFP** indicates an open neural tube defect, a multiple gestation, a ventral (abdominal) wall defect, inaccurate dates → while a **decreased AFP** is Down syndrome, inaccurate gestational dates, and fetal demise. An abnormal AFP should be followed with an **ultrasound** (to check dates and fetal abnormality), and then an **amniocentesis** (to check chromosomal abnormality and amniotic fluid AFP level; there is risk of fetal loss and hemorrhage with amniocentesis). **Amniocentesis is also an indication** in **pregnant women > 35 years of age**, assessing 3rd trimester **fetal lung maturity**, and in **Rh-sensitized pregnancy** (to check fetal blood type or hemolysis).

3. **By week 24-28**: Screen for diabetes with one-hour glucose tolerance test (fasting serum glucose) after an oral glucose load. The result is abnormal if $\geq$ 140 mg/dL; order a three-hour glucose tolerance test. **Recheck H/H** (hemoglobin/hematocrit) for anemia. Give **Rhogam** injection to Rh negative patients. Educate patients to start **fetal kick counting** (at least 10 fetal movements in less than an hour).

4. **By week 35-37**: Screen for **group B streptococcus** (GBS) with a rectovaginal swab. Recheck for chlamydia, gonorrhea, anemia (with H/H); and obtain RPR and HIV tests in high-risk patients. Obtain fetal ultrasound to assess fetal lie/position using **Leopold maneuvers**. Treat positive GBS with ampicillin during labor and after delivery.

5. Check fetal heart beats with Doppler at 10-12 weeks, fundal height in centimeters starting at week 20 (consider intrauterine growth restriction or retardation when

there is > 2-3 cm difference in measurement and confirm with an ultrasound), weight gain, vitals, and evaluate extremities for edema.

6. Give prenatal vitamins, iron and folate supplementation, and advice on smoking cessation.

Assessing Fetal Well-Being

1. **Nonstress test (NST)**: **normal/reactive** test includes two accelerations of 15 beats per minute above baseline more than 15 seconds and lasting over 20 minutes span. An **abnormal/nonreactive** test may be as a result of fetal sleep cycle, maternal drug use, and fetal neurological abnormality.

2. **Contraction stress test (CST)**: evaluates uteroplacental dysfunction by providing stimulations. **Normal/negative** test indicates **fetal well-being** and shows **no late decelerations**; while an **abnormal/positive** test shows **late decelerations**.

3. **Biophysical profile (BPP)**: using an ultrasound, it measures nonstress test, amniotic fluid index, fetal body movements, and fetal breathing movements. A normal test is a **negative test** with **score 8-10 (indicates fetal well-being)** and an abnormal test is a **positive test** with **score < 6** (may be due to fetal compromise).

4. **Normal fetal heart rate** is 110-160 beats per minute (bpm). **Fetal heart strip** may show **early deceleration** (begins and stops when uterine contracts) due to head compression from vagal response; this is not worrisome. A **variable deceleration** (variable in association with uterine contractions), due to umbilical cord compression, and a **late deceleration** (decelerations occur **after** uterine contractions) is **due to uteroplacental insufficiency/fetal hypoxia; this is worrisome** as it indicates **fetal distress** → **deliver fetus** if repetitive late decelerations or may initiate management by placing mother on lateral decubitus position, stop oxytocin, administer oxygen and magnesium sulfate; and assess the fetal scalp pH (if < 7.2, deliver fetus; if > 7.2, observe and deliver if needed).

Complications During Pregnancy

1. **Hyperemesis gravidarum** => 1st trimester recurrent nausea and vomiting that leads to dehydration, electrolyte imbalance, and weight loss → ask for stressors which may be contributing to this condition → risk factors that may be contributory are multiple gestation, nulliparity, and trophoblastic disease → diagnosis: electrolytes (shows hypokalemic, hypochloremic metabolic alkalosis, hyponatremia), urinalysis (ketones indicate starvation) → treatment is

supportively with antiemetic therapy, hydration, and small frequent meals; however, if symptoms are severe with electrolyte abnormality, hospitalize the patient and treat supportively.

2. **Gestational diabetes**: defined as diabetes occurring during pregnancy → risk factors include prior history of diabetes mellitus, family history in a first-degree relative, **pregestational diabetes**, and obesity. **Diagnosis**: one-hour glucose tolerance test (fasting serum glucose) after an oral glucose load with **glucose ≥ 140 mg/dL**; order a three-hour glucose tolerance test with at least **two increased levels**. **Treatment**: diabetic diet, safe-pregnancy exercise, and insulin. **Complications**: macrosomia, fetal hypoglycemia, shoulder dystocia (birth trauma), spontaneous abortion, polyhydramnios, preterm labor, preeclampsia, neural tube defects, still-birth, caudal regression syndrome (incomplete formation of the lower part of the body), and respiratory distress syndrome.

3. **Maternal hyperthyroidism**: most common cause is Grave's disease. Signs & symptoms include heat intolerance, weight loss, tachycardia/palpitations, tremor, sweating +/- goiter. **Diagnosis**: low TSH and increased free T4. **Treatment**: **propylthiouracil** (PTU) and surgery (thyroidectomy) in refractory or non-compliant patients. Complication: thyrotoxicosis (treat supportively and with PTU and propranolol).

4. **Preeclampsia**: defined as hypertension > 140/90 (**mild**), proteinuria of 1+ on dipstick or > 300 mg on 24-hour urine, lower extremity and/or facial edema, oliguria, headaches, blurry vision, and HELLP (**h**emolysis, **e**levated **l**iver enzymes, **l**ow **p**latelets) syndrome on two separate prenatal visits. **Risk factors** include African-American, nulliparity, multiple gestations, chronic hypertension, chronic renal disease, and diabetes. **Diagnosis**: 24-hour urine for protein and creatinine clearance, urinalysis, CBC, BUN, creatinine, LFTs, PT/PTT, uric acid, and fibrinogen. **Treatment**: deliver if patient is near term; but if not, manage supportively with **bed rest** and **magnesium sulfate** (for seizure prophylaxis).

5. **Severe preeclampsia**: > 160/110, proteinuria of 3+ on dipstick or > 5 g on 24-hour urine. **Treatment**: hydralazine or labetalol and magnesium sulfate (for seizure prophylaxis). When patient is stable, deliver the baby. **Eclampsia**: is defined as preeclampsia + **seizures**. **Treatment**: magnesium sulfate (to **control** seizure). When patient is stable, deliver the baby. Complications: fetal distress, fetal or maternal death.

6. **Third-trimester bleeding**: defined as bleeding after 20 weeks → causes include abruptio placentae, placenta previa, and uterine rupture. Other causes are bloody show, preterm labor, trauma, and vasa previa.

7. **Abruptio placenta**: placenta separates from its location; due to hypertension, cocaine use, trauma, polyhydramnios, and preterm premature rupture of membranes → presents as abdominal pain with increased uterine contractions,

vaginal bleeding, and fetal distress → diagnosis: ultrasound → treatment: immediate delivery (if severe) or supportively (with admission if mild).

8. **Placenta previa**: placenta is covering the os; due to prior c-section, prior placenta previa, and multiple gestations → presents as painless vaginal bleeding usually without uterine contractions and without fetal distress → diagnosis: ultrasound → treatment: serial ultrasounds (for monitoring previa status) +/- c-section (for partial or total placental previa).

9. **Uterine rupture**: due to previous uterine surgery or scar, trauma, oxytocin, multiple gestation, polyhydramnios, and grand multiparity → presents as **sudden onset of severe abdominal pain**, hypotension, shock, **fetal distress**, and look for change in the shape/outline of the abdomen → diagnosis: clinical → treatment: **immediate laparotomy or c-section +/- hysterectomy after delivery**.

Abnormal Labor and Delivery

1. **Preterm labor**: labor that occurs between 20-37 weeks of gestation → Findings: abdominal/pelvic pain, pelvic pressure, back pain, uterine contractions (look for cervical change with more than 3 contractions which last for 30 seconds and over a 30-minute period that occurs **before 37 weeks of gestation**), vaginal discharge +/- bleeding → diagnosis: ultrasound (check fetal presentation and amniotic fluid) → treatment: **IVFs, bed rest with lateral decubitus position, oxygen +/- steroids** and **tocolytics**. Consider GBS prophylaxis. Complications include intraventricular hemorrhage, fetal respiratory distress syndrome, or fetal death.

2. Preterm premature rupture of membranes (PPROM): premature rupture of the membranes **at < 37 weeks before the onset of labor** → risk factors include smoking, STDs, and low socioeconomic status → diagnosis: culture and gram stain → treatment: antibiotics (amoxicillin) if positive for infection; or if negative, bed rest, hydration, follow-ups +/- steroids (for lung maturity).

3. Premature rupture of membranes (PROM): rupture of the membranes **at term (> 37 weeks)** but before the onset of labor → leading to loss of fluid → diagnosis: **sterile speculum exam** (shows **pooling of amniotic fluid, nitrazine paper test** turns blue in alkaline amniotic fluid, **fern test** shows ferning pattern under microscope and allowed to dry), and **ultrasound** (assess amniotic fluid volume, gestational age, and congenital abnormalities) → treatment: ampicillin (covers amnionitis) +/- gentamicin; labor should follow after PROM; if not, **induce labor**.

4. **Genital herpes** in an indication for cesarean section (if there are active lesions during labor and patient has been noncompliant with acyclovir therapy which is usually started at 36 weeks) → risk of delivering via vaginal can lead to eye

infections.

5. **Shoulder dystocia** => occurs as a result of arrest disorder/failure to progress during labor and delivery → risk factors: macrosomia, prior history of shoulder dystocia, or inadequate pelvis → diagnosis: 2nd stage labor is prolonged where the head is retracted back into the vaginal cavity (known as the turtle sign) and the **anterior shoulder is difficult to deliver** after the head is already out → manage with **McRobert maneuver** where the mother flexes her thigh against her abdomen to free the impacted shoulder, apply **suprapubic pressure**, then **deliver the posterior fetal arm** by **internal rotation** of the shoulders. This should deliver the fetus. However, if no progress, replace the fetal head back into the vaginal cavity, and perform a c-section (this is known as **Zavanelli maneuver**).

6. **Fetal malpresentation** => for shoulder or footling presentation, deliver via c-section → for face/brow (vertex) presentation, watchful waiting and deliver via vaginal.

7. **Do not induce or augment labor in these conditions:** previous cesarean section incision, vasa previa, placenta previa, transverse fetal lie, umbilical cord prolapsed, genital herpes, or cervical cancer → management: deliver via c-section.

8. **Indication for cesarean section:** previous cesarean section, cephalopelvic disproportion, genital herpes, placenta previa, placental abruption, cervical cancer, fetal malrepresentation, fetal distress, and erythroblastosis fetalis.

9. A previous vertical uterine incision for c-section is an indication for **future c-sections** (to prevent uterine ruptures) → however, a previous low segment, horizontal, uterine incision may be followed with future vaginal deliveries.

Postpartum Complications

1. **Postpartum hemorrhage**: defined as > 500 ml of blood loss during a vaginal delivery or > 1000 ml of blood loss during a cesarean section. The **most common cause** is **uterine atony**; and others include retained placental tissue (placenta accrete, increta, percreta), lacerations/genital tract trauma, uterine inversion, coagulation disorders (DIC, von Willebrand disease), and low placental implantation.

2. **Uterine atony**: most commonly due to **overdistention of the uterine** (due to polyhydramnios, multiple gestation), **prolonged labor** (resulting in uterine infection), **use of oxytocin** (most common), and grand multiparity (history of many vaginal deliveries > 5) → diagnosis: palpation of **soft, enlarged, "boggy"**

uterus → treatment: **vigorous bimanual compression** and **massage** of the uterus with **oxytocin infusion** +/- ergonovine (methylergonovine, if no response to other treatment or hypertensive), prostaglandin F2-alpha (not indicated if asthmatic), or misoprostol. Hysterectomy may be considered if there is severe bleeding.

3. **Retained placental tissue**: due to placental tissue (placenta accrete, increta, percreta), **prior c-section, prior uterine surgery**, retained membranes → diagnosis: ultrasound (shows retained placenta) and **inspection of the uterine cavity** and **placenta** → treatment: **manually remove the placenta** (helps to stop the bleeding), curettage (in the OR) +/- hysterectomy (in severe bleeding).

4. **Genital tract trauma**: caused by precipitous delivery (< 3 hours), laceration, operative vaginal delivery (such as using forceps), and macrosomia → diagnosis: **inspect the cervix, vagina,** and **vulva** for any signs of trauma → treatment: surgical repair of the defect.

5. **Uterine inversion**: uterus inverts and is visualized outside of the vagina as "beefy mass" → caused by excessive pulling on the umbilical cord → treatment: **uterine replacement** by placing the uterus back in its position, IVFs, and oxytocin.

6. **Sheehan syndrome**: patients with severe postpartum hemorrhage (blood loss and hypotension) may develop postpartum hypopituitarism → due to anterior pituitary insufficiency as a result of pituitary ischemia → patients complain of **failure to lactate**, amenorrhea, anorexia, and weight loss → treatment: hydrocortisone.

7. Watch for **amniotic fluid pulmonary embolism** in a postpartum woman who develops dyspnea, chest pain, tachypnea, and hypotension.

8. **Postpartum fever**: persists for two days due to infections such as **endometritis** (due to prolonged labor, c-section, frequent vaginal exams during labor, premature rupture of membranes), urinary tract infection, breast engorgement, atelectasis, removal of retained products, and chorioamnionitis (infection **during** labor due to prolonged rupture of the membranes). **Findings: painful uterus +/- foul-smelling lochia** (common in endometritis/chorioamnionitis). For **endometritis**: diagnosis is with pelvic exam for cause, urinalysis, urine culture, CBC with differential, blood cultures, and cultures of the endometrium and vagina. Treatment is with **broad-spectrum antibiotics**; (for chorioamnionitis, deliver the baby).

9. **Mastitis:** Lactating women with tender, reddish, hard, swollen, fluctuant mass of the breast → other signs are fever and malaise → diagnosis: CBC and cultures of the breast milk → treatment: continued breast-feeding, antibiotics such as dicloxacillin/erythromycin, and NSAIDs. Complication: breast abscess (treat with incision and drainage).

Abortion
Spontaneous Abortion

1. Sudden and nonelective termination of pregnancy at < 20 weeks of gestation.
2. Findings: identify the type of spontaneous abortion seen below.
3. Diagnosis: cervical exam (to view the cervix and expulsion of products), and ultrasound.
4. Treatment: check patient for bleeding and stabilize as needed, beta HCG (to confirm pregnancy), and transvaginal ultrasound (to assess fetal heartbeat and remaining products of conception). Provide Rhogam for Rh negative women.

Types of spontaneous abortion:

1. Threatened abortion: uterine bleeding which may present with some pain/cramps, **no cervical dilation**, and no expulsion of products of conception → diagnosis: cervical exam (shows closed cervical os) and ultrasound (shows gestational sac) → treatment: pelvic rest/expectant management and avoid intercourse until advised to resume.

2. Inevitable abortion: uterine bleeding **with pain/cramps, cervical dilation**, and no expulsion of products of conception → diagnosis: cervical exam (shows opened cervical os) and ultrasound (shows gestational sac) → treatment: observation, then dilatation and curettage (D&C).

3. Incomplete abortion: uterine bleeding **with pain/cramps, cervical dilation**, and **some expulsion of products of conception** → diagnosis: cervical exam (shows opened cervical os) and ultrasound (shows gestational sac) → treatment: observation, then dilatation and curettage (D&C).

4. Complete abortion: decreased uterine bleeding **with minimal pain/cramps, cervical dilation**, and **all expulsion of products of conception** → diagnosis: cervical exam (shows closed cervical os) and ultrasound (shows **vacant/empty uterus**) → treatment: obtain serial HCG and monitor until it goes down to zero; may need dilatation and curettage (D&C) if cervical os is opened and presents with pain.

5. Missed abortion: fetal death **without expulsion of products of conception** → diagnosis: cervical exam (shows closed os) and ultrasound (shows **no fetal heart tone** and evidence of fetal tissue) → treatment: products of conception (POC) may pass spontaneously within 4 weeks; otherwise, manage with **misoprostol** or D&C.

6. Septic abortion: associated with recent history of therapeutic abortion that leads to malodorous discharge → look for cervical motion tenderness on exam →

135

treatment: supportively with oxygen, IVFs, antibiotics, and D&C.

7. Induced abortion: elective and planned termination of pregnancy at < 20 weeks of gestation. Sometimes abortion is done to preserve/maintain the life of the pregnant woman.

Recurrent Abortion

1. Recurrent abortion is defined as at least three unplanned abortions or loss of pregnancies before 20 weeks of gestation.
2. Etiology: **chromosomal/uterine abnormalities**, infection (*Toxoplasmosis, Listeria, Mycoplasma*, syphilis), autoimmune (**antiphospholipid antibodies**), anatomical abnormalities (**cervical incompetence**, fibroids), diabetes, and environmental (drugs, alcohol, smoking).
3. Diagnosis: based on the clinical findings and history; pelvic exam, cervical cultures for infections, labs (TFTs, lupus anticoagulant, and anticardiolipin antibody), sonohysterogram, and genetic (chromosomal) analysis.
4. Treatment: based on diagnosis.

OBSTETRICS 1-LINER JUNKY CASES

- Normal pregnancy => absence of menstrual cycle which is confirmed with a **positive beta HCG test** → Findings: amenorrhea + **Chadwick sign** (darkening of the wall of the vagina and vulva) + nausea + vomiting + breast tenderness and fullness + **Hegar sign** + weight gain + melasma + line nigra (dark vertical line on the abdomen) → remember HCG levels double every two days in the 1st trimester → **important labs** include overall decreased hemoglobin and hematocrit (since plasma volume increases > than hemoglobin); T4 and thyroid-binding globulin increase, but free T4 is normal; increased minute ventilation (due to increased tidal volume).

- Pregnant women require the same urgency when it comes to surgery such as appendicitis and cholecystitis.

- Intrauterine growth retardation (IUGR) => risk factors include alcohol, cigarettes, drugs, hypertension, preeclampsia, TORCH (**t**oxoplasmosis, **o**thers [congenital syphilis, viruses], **r**ubella, **c**ytomegalovirus (**most common**), and **h**erpes simplex virus) infections; and congenital abnormalities → diagnosis: **ultrasound** used to determine IUGR measures head and abdominal circumferences, femur length, and biparietal diameter → treatment: includes **prevention** (smoking cessation, dietary changes, and well-controlled blood pressure) and ultrasound follow-ups to measure growth advancement → deliver at term.

- Oligohydramnios => due to IUGR, **renal agenesis**, polycystic kidneys, premature rupture of membranes (PROM) → **diagnosis: ultrasound** shows **decreased amniotic fluid** (< 300-500 ml), **amniotic fluid index (AFI) ≤ 5** cm, and ferning test (for rupture of membranes) → **treatment**: may benefit from amnioinfusion during labor (prevents umbilical cord compression) → complication: **fetal hypoxia** (due to umbilical cord compression), pulmonary hypoplasia and skeletal abnormalities (such as facial distortion).

- Polyhydramnios => due to multiple gestation, maternal diabetes, omphalocele, neural tube defects, and hydrops fetalis → **diagnosis: ultrasound** shows **increased amniotic fluid** (> 1700-2000 ml), **amniotic fluid index (AFI) ≥ 25** cm, and glucose testing (for diabetes) → **treatment**: depends on the cause → complication: preterm labor, placental abruptio, and uterine atony.

- Arrest disorder => no cervical changes over 2 hours when true labor has already begun → treat with labor augmentation such as oxytocin, prostaglandin gel, amniotomy +/- cesarean section (if no response to medication).

- Cephalopelvic disproportion => results in failure to progress due to difference in the size of the infant's head and the mother's pelvis → (do not give oxytocin to augment labor) → treatment: c-section.

- Oxytocin therapy during ineffective uterine contractions can lead to **uterine hyperstimulation, uterine rupture, water intoxication** (ADH causing hyponatremia)**, and fetal heart rate deceleration** → discontinue oxytocin.

- Prostaglandin E2 or dinoprostone is usually administered with oxytocin to enhance the ripening the cervix for induction of labor.

- General anesthesia during delivery imposes the risk of aspiration pneumonia → epidural anesthesia (not spinal anesthesia) is the best option.

- No breast-feeding with underlying HIV infection, active hepatitis infection, and while taking drugs such as warfarin, tetracycline, or chloramphenicol.

- Rhesus (Rh) isoimmunization/Rh incompatibility/hemolytic disease of the newborn => mother is Rh negative and child is Rh positive → this means the father must be Rh positive (if the father was Rh negative along with the mother, child would have been Rh negative too and no incompatibility would form) → however, because the child is Rh positive (and father must be Rh positive; child has 50% chance of being Rh positive) → due to fetal Rh positive leaking into Rh negative maternal circulation; maternal Rh IgG antibodies form and crosses the placenta to react with fetal RBCs to cause **fetal hemolysis** → **treatment: give mother Rh immune globulin** at **28 weeks and within 72 hours after delivery** and during any procedures such as amniocentesis → For hemolytic disease to occur, previous sensitization (during exposure to blood products, abortion, ectopic pregnancy, previous delivery of an Rh positive child, amniocentesis) must have occurred.

- Gestational trophoblastic disease (GTD) => cause includes **hydatiform mole** (**most common cause**, benign) or choriocarcinoma (malignant) → in **hydatiform mole, preeclampsia occur** before the third trimester or < 24 weeks, uterine size greater than gestational age/dates, HCG rapidly rises during pregnancy with **excessive nausea** and **vomiting, first-trimester bleeding, no fetal heartbeat/tone**, expulsion of **grape-like molar clusters** on pelvic exam, and "**snow storm**" pattern on ultrasound → treatment: uterine **dilatation and curettage** with follow-ups on serial beta HCG measurements until they reach zero → **choriocarcinoma** is suspected when beta HCG levels fail to decrease → obtain chest x-ray (for metastases), **chemotherapy (methotrexate** or actinomycin D) +/- hysterectomy → provide OCPs for contraception and monitoring of beta HCG levels.

- Lochia => **normal vaginal discharge** at postpartum that starts off as red, and it gradually changes color to white by day 10 after vaginal delivery → however

138

watch for foul smell which may **indicate endometritis**.

Chapter 12
Gynecology
Contraception

1. Contraception is used to prevent pregnancy (and there is no benefit for STD protection). It is also used to help regulate menstrual cycles and symptoms of fibrocystic disease. The following are the forms of contraception:
2. **Emergency contraception: A progestin-only** hormonal drug, **levonorgestrel**, which is usually administered within 72 hours of unprotected sexual intercourse and again 12 hours later in order to decrease the risk of pregnancy → it is only effective for the first 5 days after unprotected sexual intercourse.
3. **Intrauterine devices (IUDs):** The two types are **copper** and **levonorgestrel IUDs. Copper** (Paraguard) => nonhormonal, and it lasts **10 years**; recommended for patients with **less menstrual flow** and seek longer contraception; **side effects:** dysmenorrhea, pelvic pain, and increased menstrual flow. **Levonorgestrel** (Mirena) => hormonal (progesterone), and it lasts **5 years**; recommended for patients with **heavy menstrual flow with pain/dysmenorrhea** and seek longer contraception; **side effects:** amenorrhea or irregular menstrual cycles. Patients with STDs are not recommended to use IUDs for contraception.
4. **Medroxyprogesterone Acetate (Depo-Provera):** Hormonal injections given intramuscularly every 3 months for contraception → it is convenient (no everyday pills), effective, and safer for patients with history of thromboembolism → side effects include amenorrhea/oligomenorrhea and **osteoporosis** with long-term use.

Benefits of Oral Contraception Pills (OCPs)

1. Decreases ovarian cancer.
2. Decreases endometrial cancer.
3. Decreases incidence of breast disease (not breast cancer).
4. Decreases dysmenorrhea and menorrhagia.
5. Decreases dyspareunia.

Contraindications to Oral Contraception Pills (OCPs)

1. Smoking (ongoing) after the age of 35.
2. Pregnancy.
3. Uncontrolled hypertension.
4. Previous history of thromboembolism.
5. Current or undiagnosed genital bleeding.
6. Active liver disease or hepatocellular carcinoma.
7. Stroke or coronary artery disease.
8. Estrogen-dependent neoplasm.

Amenorrhea

- **Primary amenorrhea**: No presence of menstrual cycle by age 16 with secondary characteristics; or absence of menstrual cycle and secondary sexual characteristics by age 14. **Check for** breast, uterus and vagina → diagnosis: First **beta HCG (pregnancy test)** and ultrasound; if there is **breast and uterus**, differential diagnosis can be **vaginal septum, anorexia, pregnancy, imperforate hymen, or excessive exercise**. If there is **no breast** (uterus present), **order FSH and karyotype** (rule out Turner syndrome—X0 and **increased FSH;** or hypothalamic pituitary failure—XX and **low FSH**). If there is **no uterus** (breast present), order **testosterone** and **karyotype** (rule out Mullerian agenesis—XX; testicular feminization—XY; both have **normal testosterone**).

- **Secondary amenorrhea**: Absence of menstruation for six months or three cycles in a previously menstruating female → diagnosis: first, beta HCG test to rule out **pregnancy**; TSH (high; hypothyroidism), prolactin (high; hyperprolactinemia), then **progesterone withdrawal test** (if bleeding occurs after administering progesterone, progesterone is deficient=**anovulation** and estrogen is sufficient) → obtain LH level; if high, think of PCOS. If LH is low, think of **anorexia nervosa, strenuous exercise, hypothyroidism, stress, hyperprolactinemia, chronic anovulation,** or **intrauterine adhesions**.

- However, in an **estrogen-progesterone withdrawal test** (for secondary amenorrhea), if there's any bleeding at all, estrogen is deficient. Obtain FSH level. If FSH is high (> 40 mIU/mL), there may be **gonadal/premature ovarian failure** or **menopause** (associated with autoimmune disease, history of chemotheraphy, and karyotype abnormalities). If FSH is low (< 40 mIU/mL), there may be severe hypothalamic dysfunction secondary to hypothalamic neoplasm (confirm with an MRI of the brain). If there was no bleeding with the

withdrawal test (negative), there may be an anatomic abnormality due to outflow tract obstruction/adhesion; rule out asherman's syndrome by ordering **hysterosalpingogram** (shows scarring of the endometrium).
- Treatment depends on the cause of amenorrhea above. **Clomiphene** may be tried for upto 6 cycles to achieve pregnancy.

Dysmenorrhea

1. Pelvic pain associated with menstrual cycles that may interfere with daily activities.
2. **Primary dysmenorrhea**: Pain that is due to increased uterine prostaglandin production.
3. **Secondary dysmenorrhea**: Pain is usually due to an underlying condition such as adenomyosis, endometriosis, myomas, and pelvic inflammatory disease.
4. Diagnosis: Usually clinical.
5. Treatment: NSAIDs.

Abnormal Uterine Bleeding

1. It is defined as bleeding occurring with changes in menstrual flow (ovulatory) or occurring in any manner (**anovulatory**; **most common**) due to a pathology such as unopposed estrogen with increased risk of endometrial hyperplasia or endometrial cancer.
2. **Dysfunctional uterine bleeding**: Diagnosis of exclusion. It is the **most common cause of abnormal uterine bleeding** and **anovulation**. DUB may be due to infections. Treat with NSAIDs or birth control pills (OCPs).
3. Diagnosis: Initially with transvaginal speculum exam for blood, beta HCG, and CBC.
4. Treatment: Treat the underlying cause; high-dose IV estrogens, dilatation and curettage, uterine artery embolization, or hysterectomy. Treat DUB with NSAIDs or birth control pills (OCPs).
5. Other (lesser) causes of abnormal uterine bleeding are: **anatomical** such as endometrial hyperplasia, leiomyoma (check with ultrasound, hysteroscopy); **systemic** such as von Willebrand's disease, endocrine abnormalities (check with coagulation profile, TSH, FSH, LH, prolactin); **malignancies** such as endometrial and cervical (check with endometrial biopsy and papsmear with biopsy); and **postmenopausal bleeding** (check history of hormone and endometrial biopsy). Remember to rule out endometrial cancer with endometrial biopsy in women over the age of 35.

Endometriosis

1. Endometrial glands located outside the uterine lining such as in the ovaries ("**chocolate cysts/mulberry spots/powder burns**"), cul-de-sac, and broad ligament.
2. Findings: Pelvic pain, dyspareunia (pain with sexual intercourse), dysmenorrhea, and infertility. Other findings are painful nodularity along broad or uterosacral ligament, large ovaries, and retroverted uterus.
3. Diagnosis: Laparoscopy with direct visualization of endometriosis (diagnostic and therapeutic).
4. Treatment: OCPs, danazol, GnRH agonists, and surgical laparoscopy (helps to remove the endometriosis and improves infertility). If patient has completed having children, hysterectomy with bilateral salpingo-oopherectomy is the definite treatment.
5. Complication: Infertility.

Polycystic Ovarian Syndrome (PCOS)

1. PCOS is the most common cause for infertility and hirsutism in women < 30 years of age.
2. Findings: Women are obese and have abnormal hair growth (hirsutism), infertility, and **amenorrhea/oligomenorrhea**. Look for enlarged ovaries.
3. Diagnosis: Pelvic ultrasound (shows multiple ovarian cysts with follicles), increased LH:FSH > 2:1, hyperandrogenism (hirsutism/elevated testosterone), glucose level (increased; for diabetes), and **increased dehydroepiandrosterone sulfate (DHEAS)**.
4. Treatment: OCPs/cyclic progesterone (to suppress ovarian steroidogenesis), clomiphene (to induce ovulation), and weight loss +/- metformin (for insulin resistance/obesity/diabetes).
5. Complication: Endometrial hyperplasia and endometrial cancer (due to unopposed estrogen).

Vaginal Discharge & Infections

1. **Bacterial vaginosis**: Vulvovaginitis → Findings: Whitish or grayish discharge with **fishy odor** → diagnosis: Swab from the vagina, potassium hydroxide (KOH) prep which shows positive "**whiff test**" with fishy odor; pH is > 7. Saline

smear/wet moutnt is > 20% of epithelial cells (**clue cells**) → treatment: Metronidazole.
2. **Yeast (candida)**: Cottage-cheese/curdlike vaginal discharge → Findings: Irritating, pruritus/itching, erythema → diagnosis: Swab from the vagina, KOH prep shows pseudohyphae and spores; **pH is < 7** → treatment: Oral or topical antifungal.
3. **Trichomonas vaginalis**: Malodorous vaginal discharge → Findings: yellowish/greenish discharge, frothy, swollen and erythematous vagina and cervix → diagnosis: Swab from the vagina, saline smear/wet mount shows motile, flagellated protozoans; pH is > 7 → treatment: metronidazole.

Pelvic Inflammatory Disease (PID)

1. Infection of the upper genital tract usually caused by complication of either chlamydia or gonorrhea infection or both. *E. coli* has been known to cause PID also. ***Actinomyces Israeli*** is associated with intrauterine device (IUD) use. Therefore, IUD is not recommended once a patient has been diagnosed with an STD.
2. Findings: Fever +/- chills, purulent cervical discharge, dyspareunia, pelvic/abdominal pain, adnexal tenderness and cervical motion tenderness.
3. Diagnosis: CBC with differential (**elevated WBCs**), ESR, gram stain, and endocervical smear.
4. Treatment: For outpatient => use **2nd generation cephalosporin** (cefoxitin/ceftriaxone) and **doxycycline**. In patient => use clindamycin + gentamicin.
5. Complications: Tubo-ovarian abscess (usually palpable on examination), abscess rupture (**treat with emergent laparotomy**), infertility (scarring of the tubes). Note that PID is the **most common cause of preventable infertility** by using condoms.

Infertility

1. Infertility is the evidence of failed attempts to get pregnant after one year of unprotected sexual intercourse with attempts of trying to get pregnant.
2. Etiology: **Women** (50% of the cases): usually due to **tubal problems** such as PIDs or ectopic pregnancies and **uterine problems** such as endometriosis, myomas, or adenomyosis. **Other causes** are cervicitis, previous procedural biopsy (cone biopsy), ovarian failure, PCOS, prolactinemia, or birth trauma. **Men** (35% of the cases): due to spermatogenesis abnormality or varicoceles.
3. Diagnosis: **Women:** FSH, LH, TSH, prolactin, hysterosalpingography (to visualize tubal/uterine abnormalities); ovulation kits and basal body temperatures

(for ovulation dysfunction). **Men: semen analysis**.
4. Treatment: Treat the underlying cause. For endometriosis, use surgical laparoscopy (helps to remove the endometriosis and improves infertility). Clomiphene for ovulation induction.

Breast Disorders

1. **Fibrocystic disease: Most common breast disorder in women of ages 20-50** → Premenstrual, tender breasts which are usually lumpy/nodular/cystic bilaterally → **diagnosis**: clinical with physical examination; **aspiration of the cyst fluid** may be needed in women > 35 years old → **treatment**: OCPs and follow-ups for benign aspirations. Remember, there is increased risk of breast cancer with the presence of **atypia hyperplasia**.

2. **Fibroadenoma: Most common benign tumor of the female breast** → associated with changes in the menstrual cycle → presents as a painless, rubbery, unilateral mobile mass → **diagnosis**: mammogram, ultrasound, biopsy (in high-risk patients) → **treatment**: may **disappear spontaneously**; however **excision is curative**. Recurrence is common.

3. **Mastitis:** Lactating women with tender, reddish, hard, swollen, fluctuant mass of the breast → other signs are fever and malaise → diagnosis: CBC and cultures of the breast milk → treatment: continued breast-feeding, antibiotics (erythromycin), and NSAIDs.

4. **Breast abscess:** Usually a complication of breast mastitis → presents as fluctuant mass with fever, chills, and malaise → diagnosis: clinical → treatment: **surgical drainage** and antibiotics.

5. **Intraductal papilloma**: Discharge (usually bloody, but may be clear) from a single duct opening in the breast → diagnosis: mammogram; **rule-out cancer** → treatment: drainage and surgical exploration of the duct.

6. **Fat necrosis**: Look for history of trauma or ischemia → presents as firm, tender, erythema → diagnosis: mammogram and excisional biopsy (in high-risk to rule-out cancer) → treatment: NSAIDs +/- excisional biopsy.

Menopause

1. Lack of menstruation for at least 1 year after the age of 50. Other cause may be due to surgical removal of the uterus and irradiation of the ovaries.

2. Findings: Amenorrhea or menstrual irregularities, hot flashes, sweating, mood swings, sleep disturbances, depression with decreased libido, dyspareunia, atrophy vaginitis (vaginal itching, thinning and dryness), dysuria, and urinary incontinence.

3. Diagnosis: Amenorrhea for at least 1 year, **elevated FSH** (> 30 IU/L), bone density (for osteoporosis). **Estrone** (estrogen) is most associated with menopause.

4. Treatment: Oral and topical estrogen. Hormone therapy (estrogen replacement therapy, ERT) may be used in absence of uterus or combined estrogen and progesterone therapy if the uterus is still intact. Other treatment includes SSRIs (for mood swings and depression); calcium, vitamin D, bisphosphonate, calcitonin, and selective estrogen receptor modulators (SERMs) for osteoporosis.

5. Complications: Osteoporosis and heart disease.

GYNECOLOGY 1-LINER JUNKY CASES

- Ectopic pregnancy => look for pregnancy outside of the uterine cavity → risk factors include prior ectopic pregnancy, PIDs, tubal surgery, and history of DES exposure → Findings: pelvic pain +/- cervical motion tenderness and an adnexal mass, vaginal spotting or bleeding → diagnosis: increased beta HCG (but inconsistent with true pregnancy), **ultrasound** (shows lack of intrauterine pregnancy), laparoscopy (**definitive**) → treatment: monitor beta HCG with follo-ups, **methotrexate** (for asymptomatic patients with smaller pregnancies < 4 cm), and **laparoscopy** (definitive) → for **hemodynamically unstable patients** (with symptoms of shock), treat with **emergent surgery** → also, give rhogam to Rh negative patients and OCPs (for anovulation).

- Adenomyosis => endometrial glands located inside the uterus → presents as **large, boggy uterus,** dysmenorrhea, and menorrhagia → diagnosis: endometrial biopsy or D&C to rule-out endometrial cancer in women > 35 years of age → treatment: hysterectomy (curative).

- Leiomyomas (fibroids) => benign tumors which may grow due to estrogen-dependent → presents with dysmenorrhea (worse with menstrual cycle) and menorrhagia → diagnosis: pelvic ultrasound → treatment: myomectomy, uterine artery embolization, and hysterectomy (curative and recommended in cases of anemia) → remember to rule-out endometrial cancer with endometrial biopsy or D&C in women > 35 years of age.

- Stress incontinence => occurs as a result of inadequate support or function of the urethral sphincter due to weakening of pelvic ligaments → presents as loss of urine with coughing or laughing → diagnosis: history and straining test during pelvic exam → treatment: **kegel** (pelvic floor strengthening) exercise, weight loss, **pessaries**, and surgery.

- Urge incontinence => due to **involuntary detrusor muscle contractions** → look for neurology problems such as multiple sclerosis, diabetes, alzheimer's disease, or other neurological problems → diagnosis: cystometry → treatment: behavioral modification and anticholinergic medications.

- Imperforate hymen => a bulging hymen with blood in the vagina that cannot escape → treatment is surgical opening of the hymen.

- Usually **bilateral** breast discharge that are **non-bloody** (clear color) are **benign** (ask for history of drugs such as antipsychotics, OCPs, and hormonal therapies → if it is **unilateral** and **bloody**, evaluate further to **rule-out breast cancer**.

- **Premenstrual dysphoric disorder (PMS)** => symptoms occurring right before menstruation → presents as weight gain, breast swelling and tenderness, bloating, dysmenorrhea, headaches, nausea, +/- depression → diagnosis: clinical → treatment: **NSAIDs and antidepressants** (for symptoms of depression if severe). Diuretics and pyridoxine have both been shown to help too.

Chapter 13
Trauma/ER and Surgery
Trauma/ER

- In trauma, you should **start in this order (for primary/initial survey)** → **ABCDE** for management.
- A => airway → initially, you should **make sure the airway is clear** and **use cervical collar to stabilize the cervical spine/neck** in the case of trauma. If the airway is not clear, you may use **orotracheal/nasopharyngeal** airway and oxygen. If the patient is unconscious, consider **intubation +/- cricothyroidotomy** means of airway maintenance. Prompt intubation is the vital key to survival!

- B => breathing + ventilation → you should make sure the patient is breathing and airway is clear. If not, treat with **intubation +/- cricothyroidotomy**.

- C => circulation + proper hemorrhage control → look for signs of bleeding; obtain **2 large-bore needles, give packed RBCs** and **lactated Ringer's solution**.

- D => disability + focused neurologic assessment → you should assess alertness, stimuli response, and Glasgow coma scale (GCS) → < 8 (out of 15 score) usually indicates coma.

- E => exposure → by undressing the patient, assessing for any hidden bodily injuries while still keeping the patient warm and preventing hypothermia.

- After initial stabilization (and patient is able to speak), you should perform the **secondary survey** by asking the patient for medical history, medications; and assess the head, neck, chest, and abdomen for trauma and further management → obtain cervical spine x-rays, chest x-rays, pelvic x-rays, and CT scan of the head without contrast for head injuries.

Types of Burns

- Burns are categorized into chemical (from cleaning agents), electrical (from high-voltage source/lightning), or thermal (from hot water, fire) burns. Management is based on the depth and involvement of the skin as follows:

1. First-degree burns => appears as red, **painful, without blisters**, and involves **only the outermost skin layer, epidermis**. Treatment: the important thing is to avoid secondary infection by keeping the area clean, +/- pain medication, + tetanus vaccine.

2. Second-degree burns => appears as **red or white** (if deeper skin is involved), **painful, with blisters**, and involves **epidermis and dermis**. Treatment: use topical silver nitrate. May need admission to the hospital if there is significant involvement of the skin or the entire body surface area (at least 15%) + **lactated Ringer's solution + oxygen + pain medication +** tetanus vaccine.

3. Third-degree burns => appears as **dry, white, charred, nontender** (destroyed nerve endings), and involves the **entire skin layers**. Treatment: patients should be transferred to a **designated burn center** [involvement of the skin or the entire body surface area (at least 25%)]; manage with surgery + skin graft **+ lactated Ringer's solution** + tetanus vaccine. **Complication**: patients are at risk of myoglobinuria and **compartment syndrome**. Therefore, check baseline compartment pressures, and do serial follow-ups. Electrical burns are known to cause **abnormal cardiac rhythm** (obtain ECG).

Compartment syndrome:

1. A medical emergency that occurs due to muscle injury after trauma, heat exhaustion, or burn.
2. Findings: tenderness (unrelieved with medications), "**tightness or firmness of calf muscle**", cyanosis, **numbness** (paresthesia between the first and second toe is the first sign of compartment syndrome), palpable pulse at the dorsal pedal area, paresthesia, and **pain at the calf on passive movement**/passive dorsal flexion. Involves the compression of the **deep peroneal nerve.**
3. Diagnosis: clinical; **increased** compartment pressure (> 30 mmHg) with a **manometer**, and Doppler ultrasound (shows palpable pulses).
4. Treatment: **emergency fasciotomy** (decompressing the fascial spaces).
5. Complication: necrosis of muscle tissue and permanent damage of nerves.

<u>Temperature Irregulations</u>
<u>Hyperthermia</u>

- Abnormal increase in temperature that can be life-threatening → occurring within the **anterior hypothalamus**.

- Types: heat exhaustion, heat stroke, malignant hyperthermia, and neuroleptic malignant syndrome.

1. **Heat exhaustion**: mild increase in temperature (104°F) and sweating → treatment: cooling (blankets, cool water) and IVFs.

2. **Heat stroke**: severe increase in temperature (> 105°F), **confusion**, and without sweating; **risk of seizures** and rhabdomyolysis → treatment: **emergency cooling** (blankets, cool water), IVFs +/- diazepam (for seizures).

3. **Malignant hyperthermia**: due to increased levels of intracellular calcium → patient has history of halothane, **inhalation of nitrous oxide** (used during general anesthesia as an adjuvant), or succinylcholine use (usually used in surgery) and presents with high temperature (> 40°C), tachycardia, mottling skin + rigidity → labs will show hyperkalemia, hyperphosphatemia, increased creatine kinase, and lactic acidosis → treatment: IVFs and **dantrolene**.

4. **Neuroleptic malignant syndrome**: this is a complication of antipsychotic medication which is also life-threatening. Patients present with muscular rigidity, **high fever** (temperature), and sweating → labs will show **increased level of creatine phosphokinase (CPK)**, myoglobinuria → can worsen and lead to rhabdomyolysis → treatment: discontinue antipsychotics, hydration, and **dantrolene**/bromocriptine.

Hypothermia

1. Decrease in body temperature to low levels of < 95°F or < 35°C.
2. Findings: pale, confusion, and bradycardia.
3. Diagnosis: ABG, electrolytes, BUN/creatinine, and ECG (watch for cardiac irregularities, **J waves**).
4. Treatment: rewarm patients with blankets, warm IVFs and oxygen. Every patient should be rewarmed to the body temperature of at least 35°C before pronouncing them dead.

Frostbites:

- Localized skin injury due to exposure to cold and frozen air → depending on the severity, there may be pain and vesicular lesions (less severe) or numbness (more severe) → treatment: prevent refreezing; then rewarm with blankets and warm water.

GI TRAUMA

Acute Abdomen

1. Acute abdomen is a serious condition that warrants immediate attention including the possibility of a laparotomy to explore the cause.
2. Etiology: trauma, infection leading to peritonitis (such as rupture of an appendix), obstruction, perforation leading to pneumoperitoneum, and acute intestinal ischemia.
3. Findings: look for a patient with rebound tenderness that is diffuse, unintentional or involuntary guarding, and rigidity on examination.
4. Diagnosis: laparotomy with high suspicion (diagnostic and therapeutic); based on history and physical findings (usually if hemodynamically unstable, bleeding); CT scan of the abdomen with contrast may be used if patient is stable and you are unsure.
5. Treatment: laparotomy (diagnostic and therapeutic), IVFs, and antibiotics.

Bowel Obstruction

1. Abdominal pain due to twisting of the bowel.
2. The two types are: **small bowel** (may be due to adhesions from previous surgery, peptic ulcer disease) and **large bowel obstructions** (may be due to colon cancer, sigmoid volvulus, hernia, diverticulitis).
3. Findings: abdominal distention, abdominal pain, constipation, **bilous** (small bowel) or **feculent vomiting** (large bowel), and hyperactive bowel sounds.
4. Diagnosis: abdominal x-ray with air-fluid levels (supine and erect views).
5. Treatment: NPO, IVFs, NGT +/- laparotomy.

Respiratory
Flail Chest

1. Flail chest is the defect in the chest wall due to the fractures of several adjacent ribs.
2. Findings: breathing becomes labored and **paradoxically** in nature where the chest moves inward with inspiration and outward with expiration.
3. Diagnosis: clinical; history and physical exam is the key. Patient may also have pulmonary contusion due to blunt trauma to the chest.
4. Treatment: supportive initially with oxygen; then, intubation + positive end-expiratory pressure (PEEP; may be needed in patients having trouble breathing).

Tension Pneumothorax

1. **Tension Pneumothorax** is due to air that is trapped in the lungs caused by trauma.
2. Etiology: penetrating trauma, COPD, or positive end-expiratory pressure (PEEP).
3. **Findings:** look for a patient who presents with **hypotension, increased JVP, shock**, absent breath sounds, hypertympanic, or hyperresonant percussion sound on the affected side.
4. **Diagnosis**: obtain a chest x-ray (tracheal deviation **away** from the affected side).
5. **Treatment: Emergency needle thoracentesis** (effective in decompressing; placed at the anterior second intercostal space), then a **chest tube or thoracostomy tube** insertion.

Neurosurgery
Spinal Cord Compression

1. Spinal cord compression (caused by trauma or malignancy) requires immediate attention.
2. Findings: weakness, point tenderness, and positive Babinski sign.
3. Diagnosis: clinical with history and physical examination; MRI may be used after treatment with steroids to confirm.
4. Treatment: **immediate IV steroids** before MRI is done; then radiotherapy to manage metastases seen on MRI. Surgery may be needed in some cases for decompression.

Basilar Skull Fracture

1. Basilar skull fracture is a fracture involving the base of the skull as a result of trauma.
2. Findings: look for the **battle's sign** (ecchymosis can be found above the mastoid process) + **raccoon eyes** (periorbital ecchymosis) + CSF rhinorrhea (clear CSF fluid) and hemotympanum.
3. Diagnosis: CT scan of the head.
4. Treatment: supportive +/- surgery.

5. Complication: **facial palsy** → treatment: steroids.

Urology
Urethral Injury

1. Occurs as a result of pelvic fracture during trauma such as in a car accident.
2. Findings: look for ecchymosis at the perineum, blood can be seen at the urethral meatus opening, and high-riding prostate.
3. Diagnosis: **retrograde urethrogram** (not a foley catheter) and cystography.
4. Treatment: suprapubic catheter for bladder drainage and delayed surgical repair (6-10 weeks post injury).

Testicular Torsion

1. A medical emergency that involves the torsion of the spermatic cord.
2. Findings: acute onset, erythematous, swollen, tender, unilateral testicle/scrotum with an **absent cremasteric reflex**.
3. Diagnosis: Doppler ultrasound (will show diminished blood supply) of the testis.
4. Treatment: **immediate surgical evaluation** and orchiopexy. Immediate surgical evaluation is important because testicular survival decreases quickly after 6-8 hours of onset.

Orthopedic

1. Fractures may be initially negative on x-rays → still treat as fractures if there is high suspicion with symptoms → treatment usually includes avoid weight-bearing on affected area, casting, splinting, or crutches (for example in anterior cruciate ligament injury).

2. Fractures involving an **outstretched hand** during a fall occur in **fracture of the scaphoid bone** in children (leading to anatomical snuffbox tenderness) and **fracture of the Colles** in adults (leading to tenderness at the **distal** area of the radius). Treat scaphoid fracture with **thumb spica cast.**

3. Pelvic fracture: treatment is external fixation of the pelvis → if bleeding does not stop, proceed with **arterial embolization**.

4. **Open** fracture: a fracture with an 'open' skin → treatment: **open** reduction + internal fixation.

5. **Closed** fracture: a fracture with a 'closed' skin → treatment: **closed** reduction +/- casting procedure.

6. Development dysplasia of the hip (DDH): common in newborns + **palpable clunk** in a unilateral hip indicating positive Ortolani and Barlow maneuvers → treatment: refer to orthopedic surgeon.

Miscellaneous
Acid-Base Disorders

1. Respiratory acidosis => pCO_2 = increased, pO_2 = decreased, pH = decreased, HCO_3 = slightly increased, O_2 Saturation = decreased. Example is heroin (opiod) overdose → treatment is naloxone.
2. Respiratory alkalosis => pCO_2 = decreased, pO_2 = increased, pH = increased, HCO_3 = slightly decreased, O_2 Saturation = decreased/increased. Example is acute anxiety → treatment is lorazepam.
3. Metabolic acidosis => pCO_2 = slightly increased, pO_2 = slightly decreased/increased, pH = decreased, HCO_3 = decreased, O_2 Saturation = slightly decreased/normal. Example is prolonged diarrhea → treatment is hydration +/- loperamide.
4. Metabolic alkalosis => pCO_2 = slightly decreased, pO_2 = slightly decreased/increased, pH = increased, HCO_3 = increased, O_2 Saturation = slightly decreased/normal. Example is prolonged vomiting → treatment is antiemetic drugs such as phenergan.

Vitamins & Nutrition

1. Zinc deficiency => leads to alopecia, diarrhea, periorbital, and perioral dermatitis.
2. Selenium deficiency => leads to cardiomyopathy.
3. Iodine deficiency => leads to hypothyroidism.

TRAUMA/ER AND SURGERY 1-LINER JUNKY CASES

- Splenic rupture is usually due to blunt trauma to the abdomen from a motor vehicle accident (most common cause) → patient presents with LUQ tenderness, **referred pain to the left shoulder (Kehr sign)** → diagnosis: CT scan of the abdomen → treatment: surgery.
- Preferred IVFs in trauma/burn => **lactated Ringer's solution**.
- In the case of abuse (physical, child), you should proceed with medical evaluation and treatment **before** notifying the law enforcement (eg. police).
- In a patient with drug overdose in attempt of suicide → initial therapeutic attempt should include **gastric lavage**.
- Ethylene glycol (antifreeze) intoxication => causes renal failure + **oxalate crystals** in urine → treatment: **dialysis** + gastric lavage, IV ethanol, and thiamine.
- Massive hemothorax affects the 'lungs', so presents with "**decreased breath sounds**", normal heart sounds, and "**collapsed neck veins**" caused from trauma → treatment: packed RBCs, IVFs; then chest tube +/- thoracotomy (for severe bleeding).
- Cardiac tamponade => affects the '**heart**', so presents with normal breath sounds, "**muffled heart sounds**", and "**distended neck veins**" → treatment: pericardiocentesis or pericardial window.
- Hydrocele => look for 'transillumination' and processus vaginalis remnant.
- Varicocele => look for 'non-transillumination' and pampiniform venous plexus dilatation → scrotum feels like a "bag of worms."
- Epistaxis => due to trauma to the nose, nasal septal deviation, or dry nostrils → leads to bleeding in the nose →treatment: stop the bleeding by applying pressure and topical phenylephrine; then cauterization.
- Priapism => pain erection at corpus cavernosum → treatment is phenylephrine within the first 12 hours to avoid complications.
- Cystic hygroma => benign; commonly seen in Turner syndrome patients with **lymphangioma** → treatment: surgery.
- Thyroglossal duct cysts => benign cysts, which are midline, move when the tongue is protruded.
- Brachial cleft cysts => benign cysts; are located laterally to the neck.
- Anterior cruciate ligament (ACL) tear => patient complains of a '**popping**' sound after a knee injury (sports) → positive anterior drawer test where the knee/tibia is pulled forward a little too much while flexed in a 90° angle → treatment: NSAIDs + no weight-bearing + knee immobilization + ice + elevation of the leg + crutches.
- Posterior cruciate ligament (PCL) tear => positive posterior drawer test where the knee/tibia is pushed backwards a little too much while flexed in a 90° angle.
- Lateral collateral ligament injury => positive varus stress test where the ankle is **adducted** as the knee is being held in a 30° angle.

- Medial collateral ligament injury => positive valgus stress test where the ankle is **abducted** as the knee is being held in a 30° angle.
- Cervical lymphadenitis that is not responding to antibiotics should warrant tuberculosis testing with a lymph node biopsy and surgical excision of the lymph node.
- For centrally located lung mass (confirmed via chest x-ray and CT scan of the chest), management should include bronchoscopy with transbronchial biopsy.
- For abscesses, consider surgical drainage (incision and drainage; **definitive treatment**) **before** antibiotics in your management.
- Transitional cell carcinoma of the bladder (stage 1) => hematuria + history of smoking → treatment: transurethral resection + chemotherapy.
- DVT prophylaxis for pelvic surgery in perioperative period => heparin (low-molecular-weight heparin).
- Tetanus immunization requires **three doses** of tetanus immune globulins → a **booster tetanus toxoid** is then required **every ten years** → if an injury/trauma occurs, a booster tetanus toxoid is required **every five years** → if a patient has no immunization history at all, a **booster tetanus toxoid + tetanus immune globulin** are both required.
- Appendicitis => look for leukocytosis + periumbilical pain + fever → due to obstruction of appendiceal lumen + lymphoid hyperplasia.
- Appendicitis in a pregnant woman may present with 'generalized' abdominal pain → still proceed with appendectomy! → use **fluid preloading** in anesthesia to prevent hypotension → using ketamine for anesthesia may cause preterm labor.
- Incidental finding of a liver mass on CT scan => hemangioma (carvenous) → treatment: observe.
- Undescended testes (**cryptorchidism**) usually descend by 3 months of age) => treatment: **orchiopexy** (by 1 year of age) → if the child is > 3 months of age, and the testes have not descended, choose orchiopexy (not observation management) → remember, orchiopexy does not reduce the risk of testicular cancer!
- An ileus that occurred status-post laparotomy should be decompressed → use nasogastric tube, NGT for decompression.
- Abdominal pain + distention + N/V after several days of percutaneous GI tube => **paralytic ileus** → diagnosis: abdominal x-rays → treatment: nasogastric tube, NGT for decompression.
- Hypokalemia can also cause paralytic ileus.
- **Mesenteric ischemia** => look for a patient with history of DM, atrial fibrillation, and hypertension → patient will have pain that is out of proportion with findings + pain after eating → atrial fibrillation makes the patient more at risk of embolism → **superior mesenteric artery** (SMA) is affected → lab shows **metabolic acidosis (lactic acidosis)** on ABG + **leukocytosis**; may order **angiography** → or treat with surgery (**embolectomy + revascularization**).
- During an appendectomy and you find an incidental mass at the tip of the appendix (**carcinoid tumor**) → treatment: continue appendectomy only (if mass < 2cm) or perform hemicolectomy (if mass > 2cm).
- **Subclavian steal syndrome** => look for a patient who has cramping or

claudication in the arm usually after exercise + dizziness/vertigo/syncope (**neurological symptoms**) + reduced radial pulses on the same side; (**vertebral artery** is involved) → diagnosis: **arteriogram** (may show stenosis of the subclavian artery) → treatment: **carotid-subclavian bypass**.

- **Fat embolism** => confusion + petechiae after bone fracture.
- Testicular torsion => treatment: orchiopexy. (Hint: it's **p**ainful => orchio**p**exy).
- Cryptorchidism => treatment: orchio**p**exy.
- Testicular cancer => treatment: orchie**c**tomy.
- Cocaine abuse => causes vasospasm + it leads to acute myocardial infarction (MI) → treatment: nitroglycerin (NTG) + aspirin + **lorazepam**; then cardiac catherization + percutaneous angioplasty STAT!
- Stress incontinence → **overflow incontinence** → postvoid residual urine volume is usually around 200 mL → treatment: **intermittent foley catheterization** → same treatment for benign prostatic hypertrophy.
- Incontinence in neulogical disorders (multiple sclerosis) => treatment: **scheduled voiding**.
- Dementia patients with incontinence => treatment: **prompted voiding**.
- Recombinant tissue plasminogen activator (tPA) may be administered in cases of acute ischemic strokes if patients present to the emergency room within 3 hours of onset.
- Esophageal perforation => etiology is iatrogenic → look for history of endoscopy procedure that leads to **subcutaneous emphysema** → treatment: **gastrograffin contrast esophagram** + surgical repair.
- Hemorrhagic pancreatitis => continuous decrease in hematocrit + elevated WBCs (> 18K) + decreased calcium.
- Trigger finger => patient complains of pain (awakens patient) on finger when flexed + snap sound.
- De Quervain tenosynovitis occurs in a mother carrying her child in with an **extended thumb + flexed wrist**.

Chapter 14
Biostatistics

Sensitivity

- An individual **with** a disease has the probability of having a **positive** test → the number of true positives is divided by the number of people with the disease.
- Used for **screening** testing. Look for **false-positive** results.

Specificity

- An individual **without** a disease has the probability of having a **negative** test → the number of true negatives is divided by the number of people without the disease.
- Used for **confirmatory** testing. Look for **false-negative** results.

Predictive Values

1. **Positive predictive value (PPV)** => An individual with a positive result has the probability of having the disease → **true positives/all positives.** A higher PPV test = higher prevalence.
2. **Negative predictive value (NPV)** => An individual with a negative result has the probability of not having the disease → **true negatives/all negatives.** A higher NPV test = lower prevalence.
3. **Prevalence** => total number of existing cases of a disease in a population.
4. **Incidence** => number of new cases of a disease per year or occurring over a giving period of time.

How to Calculate PPV and NPV

	(+) DISEASE	(-) DISEASE
A positive test => (+)	A	B

A negative test => (-)	C	D

Calculation from the table involves:

PPV => A/(A+**B**)
NPV => D/(**C**+D)

SENSITIVITY => A/(A+**C**)
SPECIFICITY => D/(**B**+D)

NOTE: the hint to remember the formula above is to observe that only the 'B' and 'C' above swapped positions! So all you have to do is remember the top 2 or the bottom 2 formulas.

Risks

1. **Attributable risk:** risk that is measured by exposure to one risk factor.
2. **Absolute risk reduction** (ARR): absolute risk in placebo – absolute risk in patients being treated.
3. **Absolute risk:** the probability of developing a disease or risk in a time period.
4. **Relative risk (RR):** comparison of disease risk in an exposed population versus an unexposed population → RR = < 1 means the disease is not likely to be in the exposed population; and RR = > 1 means the disease is more likely to be in the exposed population. Used in **cohort** studies.
5. **Odds ratio (OR):** compares the rate of exposure among diseased and non-diseased populations. Used in **case-control** studies.

How to Calculate RR and OR

	(+) DISEASE	(-) DISEASE
A positive exposure => (+)	A	B
A negative exposure => (-)	C	D

Calculation from the table involves:

RR => [A/(A+B)]/[C/(C+D)]
OR => AD/BC

<u>Types of Studies</u>

1. **Case-control study**: Used for rare diseases → **retrospective** study involving two similar groups of people with and without a disease. They are the group of people compared to each other for exposure to risk factors. A **retrospective** study is **inexpensive, less time-consuming**, and deals with outcomes relating to past events.

2. **Cohort study**: a study based on exposure to a risk factor where a population is observed over time. Therefore, it is referred to as **observational study**. This is a prospective/follow-up study. A **prospective** study is **expensive, more time-consuming**, and deals with outcomes relating to future or present events.

3. Randomized controlled trial (RCT): **prospective** study that assigns participants to their respective groups (placebo or treatment group) and are later compared to assess whether treatment caused any changes or not. This is the **preferred study design**. It also provides a **cause-and-effect relationship**.

4. Cross-sectional study: is used to determine the prevalence of a disease/event at a single point in time.

5. Surveys => associated with subjective data reporting, and they are usually not reliable scientifically.

BIOSTATISTICS 1-LINER JUNKY CASES

- Relative risk reduction (RRR): [the event rate in controlled patients – event rate in experimental patients]/ the event rate in controlled patients.
- **Standard deviation** => 1SD = 68%, 2SDs = 95%, 3SDs = 99.7% in a normal/bell-shaped distribution.
- **Statistical significance** => p-value < 0.05 means outcome is statistically significant, and the outcome is due to random chance.
- **Confidence interval** => a confidence interval of 95% indicates 95% confidence that observed risks or odds is within the interval.
- **Number needed to treat (NNT):** NNT = 1/ARR → used to determine how many patients need to be treated in order to prevent an event.
- **Chi-squared test:** compares percentages or proportions.
- **T**-test: compares two means.
- **Analysis of variance (ANOVA):** compares three means or more.
- Remember in order to calculate predictive values, you will be given prevalence.
- Watch for **lead time bias** in screening tests. Lead time bias will be responsible for causing the increase of the length of time from diagnosis to death.

Chapter 15
Neurology
Seizures

- Febrile seizures: seizures that are caused by fever and occur between 9 months and 5 years of age → 2 types are **simple:** (short generalized seizure lasting 15 minutes without residual focal neurological deficit); treat by identifying source of fever → **complex:** (long focal seizure lasting longer than 15 minutes **with some focal neurological deficit**; treat with acetaminophen and order CBC, blood cultures, electrolytes, urinalysis, EEG, MRI, lumbar puncture.

- Absence seizures: patients have brief staring episodes with rapid blinks of the eyelids that last 5-15 seconds → diagnosis: ECG shows generalized, 3-Hz spike and wave pattern → treatment: Ethosuximide or valproate.

- Grand mal seizures: a generalized type of seizure causing sudden loss of consciousness, jerking of the muscles, biting of the tongue, lip smacking, loss of control of the posture, abnormal extension of the upper, lower extremities, back, +/- incontinence. Note that after a seizure, patients may experience **Todd's paralysis** which presents as a focal neurological deficit in the form of a stroke/TIA and resolves quickly.

- **Status epilepticus**: is described as sudden and prolonged/multiple seizures lasting **longer than 30 minutes**. It can result from rapid withdrawal of treatment from an epileptic patient → treatment: benzodiazepine (**lorazepam**), then **phenytoin, +/- phenobarbital** if seizure persists. Lorazepam may be repeated during management.

Partial seizures: two types are simple partial and complex partial seizures.

1. Simple partial seizures: presents with jerking from **one limb** to the other (**jacksonian march or seizure**) and **normal consciousness**. Look for a patient with stiffness of one extremity, then jerking + twitching + no other symptoms. It may involve the motor cortex or one of the two cerebral hemispheres. Remember to order an EEG and electrolytes.

2. Complex partial seizures: similar to simple partial seizures, but with **abnormal consciousness** affecting the temporal lobes.

Strokes

1. Ischemia resulting in neurological deficit caused by the occlusion of a large cerebral vessel (**ischemic strokes; most common, majority**) or rupture of a small vessel/**berry aneurysm (intracranial hemorrhage**).
2. Etiology: atherosclerosis resulting in ischemia, atrial fibrillation resulting in thrombosis and emboli to the brain, and endocarditis resulting in septic embolic.
3. Risk factors: atherosclerosis, hyperlipidemia, hypertension, diabetes mellitus, cigarette smoking, coronary artery disease, a recent myocardial infarction, and use of birth control pills.
4. Findings: Depends on the part of the brain being affected → **anterior cerebral artery lesion**: results in leg paresis → **posterior cerebral artery lesion**: results in homonymous hemianopia with macular sparing and patients cannot recognize familiar faces (prosopagnosia) → **superior MCA stroke**: results in opposite side (contralateral) hemisensory deficit and hemiparesis involving the face, arm, hand with facial drooping; involvement with the dominant hemisphere results in **Broca's aphasia** where patients have **nonfluent speech, poor repetition**, but good auditory comprehension → **inferior MCA stroke**: results in opposite side (contralateral) homonymous hemianopia, apraxia, and neglect of contralateral extremities; involvement with the nondominant hemisphere results in **Wernicke's aphasia** where patients have **fluent speech only (poor repetition and auditory comprehension**).
5. Diagnosis: CT scan of the head **without contrast**, TTE/**TEE** (preferred), MRI, MRA, lipids, serum glucose, HbA1c, CBC, and electrolytes.
6. Treatment: Supportively with ABCs, oxygen, IVFs, antihypertensive drugs, **aspirin** (or **clopidogrel** if already on aspirin at time of stroke), and **thrombolytics** (restrictions require the use **only within three hours of symptoms onset**).
7. Patients with **> 70% stenosis** found on MRA, may be treated with **elective carotid endarterectomy (CEA)** post-stroke. Patients with **< 70% stenosis** may be managed with **aspirin +** antihypertensive medications.

Transient Ischemic Attack (TIA)

1. Known as a 'small stroke' because it lasts from few seconds to minutes; however, it may progress for few hours before it resolves spontaneously. It can also be an indication for a future stroke.
2. Findings: unilateral hemiplegia, hemiparesis, and **amaurosis fugax** (ipsilateral blindness).
3. Diagnosis: carotid duplex ultrasound scan (shows stenosis/occlusion) and MRA.

4. Treatment: aspirin, clopidogrel, and elective carotid endarterectomy (CEA) if carotid stenois is > 70%. If stenosis < 70%, aspirn alone may be used.

Thrombolytics Criteria/Restrictions

Do not use thrombolytics when:

1. Acute intracranial hemorrhage.
2. Recent head trauma in the last three months.
3. Myocardial infarction in the last three months.
4. Major surgery in the last two weeks.
5. History of prior intracranial hemorrhage.
6. Uncontrolled hypertension
7. Lumbar puncture procedure completed in the last one week.
8. Pregnancy.

Headaches

1. **Migraine**: occurs mostly in females with peak age onset of 20 → look for positive family history (50%) → presents with recurrent, unilateral headaches, **nausea, vomiting, aura, photophobia**; may interfere with patients daily activities and cause neurological symptoms such as weakness and unilateral paresthesias. Treat with NSAIDs (initially), sumatriptan, and beta blockers (for prophylaxis).

2. **Tension headache**: most common type with peak age onset of 20 → look for **stressors in patient's life, band-like tightness at occipital** region. Treat with stress management/relaxation therapy, NSAIDs, or acetaminophen.

3. **Cluster headache**: occurs mostly in males with peak age onset of 20 → appears in 'clusters', severe, unilateral, periorbital with lacrimation, nasal congestion, and conjunctival injection → associated with Horner's syndrome. Treat with **100% oxygen** and steroids.

4. Pseudotumor cererbri: seen mostly in young, obese women → associated with consumptions of **vitamin A** and tetracycline → presents with headaches that are **worse in the mornings**, nausea, vomiting, intracranial hypertension, and papilledema → diagnosis: **normal CT scan or MRI**; lumbar puncture (shows **increased opening pressure**) → treatment: weight loss, **repeated lumbar punctures** (helps to reduce intracranial pressure), or **shunt**. Complication: **blindness**.

5. Obtain CT scans when headaches appear severe and prolonged than previous headaches.

Subarachnoid Hemorrhage

1. Etiology: rupture of **berry aneurysm** or trauma.
2. Findings: patient describes headache as the **"worst headache of my life."**
3. Diagnosis: For trauma: CT scan of the head without contrast (initially), lumbar puncture (done later; shows blood in CSF). For non-trauma, => cerebral angiogram (shows rupture of berry aneurysm).
4. Treatment: Supportive management.

Epidural Hematoma

1. Bleeding from a head trauma as a result of a temporal skull fracture and tearing of the **middle meningeal artery**.
2. Findings: headache, nausea, vomiting, hemiparesis, fixed & dilated pupil, and **lucid interval**.
3. Diagnosis: CT scan of the head without contrast (helps to visualize the bleeding; shows **biconvex lens-shaped** area).
4. Treatment: Neurosurgery consult (to stop & evacuate blood).

Subdural Hematoma

1. Bleeding that originates from a blunt trauma to the head as a result of the rupture of **bridging veins**. Commonly found in alcoholics and elderly patients.
2. Findings: headache, nausea, hemiparesis, and confusion.
3. Diagnosis: CT scan of the head without contrast (shows **cresent-shaped, concave** area).
4. Treatment: Neurosurgery consult (to stop & evacuate blood).

Multiple Sclerosis

1. Demyelinating disorder that affects mostly women between 20-40 years of age.

2. Findings: muscular weakness/paresthesia, numbness, optic neuritis leading to diminished vision and pain, diplopia, **urinary incontinence/urgency**, vertigo, **gait abnormality**, increased sensitivity, **afferent pupillary defect (Marcus Gunn pupil**—pupil dilates due to a light stimulus and delayed conduction), intranuclear ophthalmoplegia, and positive Babinski sign.
3. Diagnosis: **MRI with and without contrast** (shows demyelination plaques), CSF (shows **increased IgG/oligoclonal bands** and **myelin basic protein**), and **visual evoked potentials** (shows delayed conduction).
4. Treatment: steroids (acute exacerbations), interferons, glatiramer acetate, and baclofen (helps spascity).

Myasthenia Gravis

1. Autoimmune disorder where the antibodies destroy acetylcholine receptors at the neuromuscular junction. Most common in women between 20-40 years of age.
2. Findings: patients complain of being **'tired' toward the end of the day**, **ptosis**, **diplopia**, and **respiratory failure** (indicates crisis).
3. Diagnosis: tensilon test (demonstrated by improvement of muscle weakness after injection of a short-acting anticholinesterase, **edrophonium**), ice pack test (for ptosis), serum acetylcholine receptor antibodies, electrodiagnostic test (**repetitive nerve stimulation**), and **single fiber electromyography** (most sensitive).
4. Treatment: **pyridostigmine** (long-acting antiacetylcholinesterase), steroids/azathioprine, **plasmapheresis** (for crisis), and **thymectomy**.

Parkinson Disease

1. Parkinson's disease is due to loss of dopaminergic neurons in the **substantia nigra**. Occurs mostly in men with mean age of onset being 60.
2. Findings: slow movement/walking, **cogwheel rigidity** (muscular rigidity), mask-like face, shuffling gait, and **resting tremor.**
3. Diagnosis: clinical.
4. Treatment: **levodopa**, bromocriptine/pergolide, amantidine, trihexyphenidyl, benztropine, and surgical pallidotomy.

Dementia

1. Chronic, **irreversible** process with normal consciousness.
2. Etiologies: **Alzheimer's disease**, vascular dementia, alcoholism, or Huntington's

disease.

3. Findings: recent memory loss/impaired, inability to complete daily activities/tasks.
4. Diagnosis: reversible causes of dementia may be followed by ruling out vitamin B12 deficiency, syphilis (VDRL), normal pressure hydrocephalus, and endocrine abnormalities (TSH). Perform complete neurological examination +/- mini mental status examination.
5. Treatment: treat the underlying cause. Medications may include donepezil and memantine.

- **Delirium**:

Frequently seen in hospitalized elderly patients with **acute flunctuations** (waxing and weaning effect during the day) in consciousness mimicking a psychological problem → look for change in medications, electrolyte imbalances, or infections. **Sundowning** may be seen in patients in the hospital due to adjustment to new environment. Remember to give alcoholics **thiamine** when they present with delirium, ataxia, nystagmus, ophthalmoplegia, and confusion.

Guillain-Barre Syndrome

1. Guillain Barre Syndrome is associated with the history of a recent upper respiratory or GI (*Campylobacter jejuni*) infection.
2. Findings: symmetrical lower extremity weakness ascending to the face, paralysis, numbness, paresthesias/**decreased sensation**, and **absent deep tendon reflexes**, and respiratory failure (complication).
3. Diagnosis: **lumbar puncture** (CSF shows **increased protein** and normal WBCs = albuminocytologic), **nerve conduction study** (shows slow velocity with conduction block, denervation), CBC (shows increased WBCs), and spirometry.
4. Treatment: Protect airway (intubation), IV immunoglobulin (IVIG), plasmapheresis, spirometer (to monitor inspiratory effort), and physical therapy.

Amyotrophic Lateral Sclerosis (ALS)

1. A disabling and degenerative disease affecting both upper motor neurons (UMNs) and lower motor neurons (LMNs). Occurs mostly in men between 55-60 years of age.
2. Findings: [spasticity, positive Babinski sign, and hyperreflexia (UMNs)] and [atrophy, tongue fasciculations, flaccidity, proximal muscle weakness, and

dysarthria. **Sensation is intact**.
3. Diagnosis: EMG (shows denervation) and muscle biopsy (neurogenic atrophy).
4. Treatment: supportively; however, there is no cure. Riluzole (glutamate release antagonist; symptomatic relief only).

Vertigo
Meniere Disease

1. Cause of hearing loss in adults.
2. Findings: nausea/vomiting, ringing in the ear (tinnitus), vertigo, and hearing loss.
3. Treatment: meclizine (antihistamine).

Benign Positional Vertigo (BPV)

1. This is a benign vertigo triggered by the change in body position (such as in head movement or moving from supine to standing position) → last **less than a minute** and **resolve spontaneously**.
2. Findings: vertigo + nystagmus only (**NO hearing loss, tinnitus,** or **loss of consciousness**).
3. Treatment: avoid triggering positions. Vertigo usually resolves on it own.

NEUROLOGY 1-LINER JUNKY CASES

- Myoclonic seizures => look for multiple shock-like jerks in the body.
- Cysticercosis => causes seizures due to *Taenia solium* (pork tapeworm) infection → common in AIDs patients and immigrants from South America → diagnosis: CT scan shows ring enhancing lesions/calcifications → treatment: praziquantel.
- A CT scan can be negative **24 hours after a stroke** → start antiplatelet medications such as **aspirin** or **clopidogrel** (IF the patient was already on aspirin at the time of stroke).
- Spinal cord compression (caused by trauma or malignancy) requires treatment with IV steroids.
- Basilar skull fracture → look for the **battle's sign** (ecchymosis can be found above the mastoid process) + **raccoon eyes** (ecchymosis can be found around the eyes) + CSF rhinorrhea (clear CSF fluid) and hemotympanum.

Chapter 16
Psychiatry and Ethics
Child Psychiatry

1. **Attention-deficit hyperactivity disorder (ADHD)**: Occurs before the age of seven, but may progress on to adulthood. Look for a child who is unable to pay attention, hyperactive, or impulsive at school, home, and/or work (in adults).

2. **Autistic Disorder**: a child with social interaction impairment, repetitive behavior and restricted activities (such as head banging), poor/delayed communication that may appear to be 'babbling' words. Associated with **congenital rubella**. **Asperger's disorder** → children have **normal** language.

3. **Rett's disorder**: Mostly in girls who present with impaired language and social interaction, poor gait, and abnormal movement of the body/extremities.

4. **Oppositional defiant disorder**: Occurs mostly in males for at least **six months**. Patients are hostile with negative, defiant attitude toward members of authority (such as the police). **Conduct disorder** → patients are more aggressive without the care of others and **violating their rights**, destroying properties, bullying others, and torturing animals.

Drugs-Related & Substance Abuse
Alcohol Abuse

1. Alcohol abuse is most common in men with a prevalence of 20%; and in women with a prevalence of 10% → a positive family history increases its risk.
2. **Alcohol intoxication**: (can be life-threatening) presents with slurred speech, blackouts, ataxia, disinhibition, and coma.

3. **Alcohol withdrawal**: (can be life-threatening) presents initially and acutely (in the first 12-48 hours after the last drink) with tachycardia, seizures, tremors, and sweating. Then there may be hallucinations +/- illusions without confusion or autonomic symptoms. Finally, **delirium tremens (DTs)** occurs with the last drink by day 2-4 with hallucinations, illusions, confusion and autonomic symptoms (tachycardia and sweating) → **treatment**: admission + **benzodiazepines (lorazepam)**. Taper the dose over several days. Or begin with

a benzodiazepine taper (chlordiazepoxide). Remember to give **thiamine** before glucose when required. Watch for DTs in patients who become delirious 24 hours after surgery due to alcohol withdrawal as this can be life-threatening. Hospitalization is required if not already in a hospital. Recommend individual or group therapy.

4. **Complications**: Wernicke's encephalopathy (ataxia, confusion, and ophthalmoplegia without confabulation) and Korsakoff's syndrome (includes confabulation).

Benzodiazepines

1. Benzodiazepine intoxication (can be life-threatening) presents with drowsiness and respiratory depression → treatment: **flumazenil**.
2. Benzodiazepine withdrawal (can be life-threatening) presents with **tremors, seizures, rebound anxiety, tachycardia, +/- cardiovascular arrest** → treatment: admission + **benzodiazepines**.
3. Remember, the use of benzodiazepines + alcohol = **CNS depressants**. The same applies to **barbiturates**. They act similarly to benzodiazepines.

Opiods

1. Opiods intoxication (can be life-threatening) presents with nausea, vomiting, euphoria, drowsiness, miosis, **constipation, pupillary constriction**, and **CNS or respiratory depression** → treatment: **naloxone or naltrexone**.

2. Opiods withdrawal presents with **pupillary dilation, rhinorrhea,** anxiety, insomnia, **diaphoresis, diarrhea,** stomach cramping, and **yawning** → treatment: **methadone** (long-acting opiod).

Other Substance Abuse Drugs

1. **Marijuana**: presents with **conjunctival injection**, time distortion (slow sense of time), **amotivational syndrome**, impaired judgment, **increased cravings/appetite**, anxiety, paranoia, social withdrawal, and hallucinations.

2. **Amphetamines**: Look for psychotic symptoms, **psychomotor agitation, pupillary dilation,** tachycardia, impaired judgment, hypertension, and

hallucinations → treatment: **haloperidol** for severe agitation. **Withdrawal symptoms** may include depression, suicidal thoughts, and increased sleeping.

3. **Cocaine**: presents with hypertension, sweating, insomnia, anxiety/aggressiveness, **formications: patients feel like 'bugs crawling on their skin'**, psychosis, **heart attack,** and **stroke.** Commonly used by bipolar patients.

4. **Lysergic acid diethylamide (LSD)**: Also associated with **mushrooms** → presents with anxiety, **visual hallucinations, flashbacks, delusions,** depression, pupillary dilation, diaphoresis, and mydriasis → no withdrawal symptoms → treatment: **benzodiazepine** or antipsychotics for severe symptoms.

5. **Phencyclidine (PCP)**: violence, vertical or horizontal nystagmus, **aggressive behavior, confusion, agitation + psychosis,** and ataxia. Patients may have schizophrenia-type symptoms → there is risk of respiratory depression and coma → no withdrawal symptoms → treatment: supportive management.

6. **Caffeine**: presents with insomnia, restlessness, muscle twitching +/- arrhythmias → withdrawal symptoms include headaches, fatigue, weight gain, and irritability.

Anxiety Disorders
Panic Disorders

1. Usually seen in women around the age of 20-40 with **agoraphobia** (fear of leaving the house or being in public places alone).
2. Findings: Panic attacks with fear of dying, shortness of breath, dizziness, chest pain, palpitations, diaphoresis, nausea, and anxiety.
3. Diagnosis: Recurrent panic attacks and extreme anxiety.
4. Treatment: SSRIs, benzodiazepines (second-line due to side effect of sedation), MAOIs, or TCAs and cognitive-behavioral therapy (CBT).

Generalized Anxiety Disorder (GAD)

1. Anxiety-related to multiple areas of patient's life.
2. Findings: Excessive worry and anxiety about everything and events occurring in patient's life.
3. Diagnosis: At least **six months** of anxiety and worry about everything. Other

symptoms include insomnia, fatigue, and irritability.
4. Treatment: SSRIs, venlafaxine, buspirone (**non-sedating**), benzodiazepines (sedatitng, tolerance and dependence), TCAs, and psychotherapy.

Post-traumatic Stress Disorder (PTSD)

1. History of a life-threatening or traumatic (fatal/non-fatal) event with recurrences of the events relived through nightmares or flashbacks persisting **> 1 month**.
2. Findings: Patient experiences recurrences of traumatic events such as rape, war, violence, trauma, or natural disasters while trying to avoid thinking about them. Patient may also have been only a witness to a traumatic event to have PTSD. If others were involved, patients may feel helpless with fear. Other symptoms are depression, substance abuse, survival guilt, and anxiety.
3. Diagnosis: Recurrence of a traumatic event that persist for **> 1 month**. Look for nightmares, flashbacks, anxiety, irritability, depression, insomnia, or hypersomnolence.
4. Treatment: SSRIs (initially), TCAs, or MAOIs. Antipsychotics (risperidone), anticonvulsants (topiramate), and beta blockers (propranolol) can also be used. Cognitive behavioral therapy and group therapy are also effective.
5. **Acute Stress Disorder:** may present exactly like PTSD but occurs in **< 1 month.**
6. **Adjustment disorder with anxiety**: Usually there is anxiety and an underlying stressor the patient is trying to adjust to.

Obsessive-Compulsive Disorder (OCD)

1. Recurrent thoughts, impulses, behavior, or images occurring mostly in early adolescents to early adulthood.
2. Findings: Patients have recurrent thoughts, impulses, behavior, or images that impact their lives. Look for a patient with fear of contamination and therefore washes hands numerous times a day and repetitive routines that are time-consuming.
3. Diagnosis: Look for signs of obsessions (persistent thoughts, impulses, or images) and compulsions (repetitive behaviors) that are time-consuming (may take hours) and causing dysfunction in the life of a patient.
4. Treatment: SSRIs (**fluvoxamine**), clomipramine, and behavioral therapy (exposure technique).

Phobias

1. Types are: social, specific, and agoraphobia.
2. Findings: Social phobia => recurrent fear or embarrassment of participating in a social activity (such as addressing a large audience). Specific phobia => chronic fear of a situation or object (such as bugs or animals). Agoraphobia => extreme fear of being in public places.
3. Diagnosis: Symptoms occurring for at least **six months**. May trigger panic attacks.
4. Treatment: Treat social phobia with cognitive behavioral therapy (CBT), SSRIs, and propranolol. Treat specific phobia with **flooding, systemic desensitization, and biofeedback**.

Somatoform Disorders

1. **Somatization disorder**: Several years of multiple complaints with **non-intentional** pain symptoms in **multiple sites/organs**. Patients have **had extensive work-ups**.

2. **Hypochondriasis**: For at **least six months,** patients have **fear**; and **believe they have a disease** although **extensive work-ups are negative**.

3. **Conversion disorder**: **Non-intentional neurological symptoms** (such as sensory loss in the lower extremities/inability to walk) caused by a trigger/stressful event.

4. **Body dysmorphic disorder**: Patient believes and imagines defects in physical appearance, so he/she seeks surgical experts.

5. **Pain disorder**: Watch for patients with pain disorders worsen by other illnesses.

Mood Disorders
Major Depression or Major Depressive Disorder (MDD)

1. Depressed mood and anhedonia that persist for **more than 2 weeks**. Depression

occurs mostly in women than in men at a ratio of 2:1.

2. Findings: **SIGECAPS** => decreased or increased **s**leep, decreased **i**nterest in things used to love (**anhedonia**), **g**uilt, decreased **e**nergy, decreased **c**oncentration, increased/decreased **a**ppetite (leading to weight gain/loss), **p**sychomotor agitation, and **s**uicidal ideation. Patients can also feel sense of **hopelessness**.

3. Diagnosis: Minimum of 5 symptoms in **SIGECAPS** persisting for at least **2 weeks** leading to impairment. Look for recent stressors (3 **Ds**) in history such as **d**eath, **d**ivorce, or **d**isease.

4. Treatment: SSRIs, electroconvulsive therapy (ECT), and psychotherapy. Treat with antidepressants for a minimum of six month before tapering off.

- **Adjustment disorder with depressed mood** => a stressful event that triggers a depressed mood. For example, look for a patient who becomes sad, cries, and wants to stay at home because of a recent loss of a job.

Bipolar Disorder

1. Mood disorder that presents with mania +/- depression occurring for one week between 20-30 years of age. There are two types: **Bipolar I** (one or more manic episodes **with impairment** including **psychosis**) and **Bipolar II** (hypomania without impairment) disorders. Mania occurs with impairment and hypomania does not.

2. Findings: Decreased need for sleep, pressured speech, grandiosity, flight of ideas or racing thoughts, sexual promiscuity, and excessive spending of money occurring for at least a week.

3. Diagnosis: Positive family history, at least three of the symptoms above, and depends on mania or hypomania episodes.

4. Treatment: **Lithium** (**for** acute mania and **depression**), anticonvulsants (valproic acid, carbamazepine), and ECT.

5. Remember to screen for bipolar disorder before initiating an antidepressant in a patient to prevent acute mania episodes or psychosis.

Indications for Electroconvulsive Therapy

1. Refractory depression.
2. Acute mania/psychosis.
3. Pregnancy.
4. Anorexia/patient with refusal to consume food or drink.

5. **Side effect: retrograde amnesia**, confusion, arrhythmia, and headache.
6. **Contraindications:** Recent stroke or myocardial infarction, and intracranial mass.

Schizophrenia

1. A psychotic disorder with age-of-onset being 15-25 years of age in men and 25-35 in women.
2. Findings: **Six months or more** of delusions, hallucinations, disorganized speech, grossly disorganized or catatonic behavior, and **negative symptoms** (flat affect, avolition, alogia, apathy).
3. Diagnosis: Patient must have at least two or more of the above symptoms for six or more months.
4. Treatment: Antipsychotic medications, psychosocial therapy, and individual and family support.
5. There is association with substance abuse and **10% of schizophrenic patients commit suicide**.
6. **Other disorders similar to schizophrenia: Brief psychotic disorder** => occurs in < 1 month with psychosis. **Schizoaffective disorder** => occurs with **psychotic symptoms** without mood disorder. **Schizophreniform disorder** => same symptoms as schizophrenia, but it occurs between 1-6 months.
7. **Positive symptoms** => include hallucinations, delusions, disorganized speech, catatonic behavior, and abnormal thought process. Patients who are married, late onset, and good support system have a good prognosis.
8. **Negative symptoms** => include flat affect, anhedonia, avolition, and alogia. Patients who are single, divorced, or widowed, early onset, and have positive family history with poor support system, have a poor prognosis.

Antipsychotic Medications & Side Effects

- **Typical antipsychotics:** dopamine receptor blockade → used for treating acute/severe agitation and psychosis → examples: **high potency (haloperidol,** fluphenazine) and **low potency (chlorpromazine,** thioridazine). The high potency drugs have **more** extrapyramidal symptoms (EPS). Other side effects are dry mouth (anticholinergic) and hyperprolactinemia.

- **Atypical antipsychotics:** act via 5HT2 and dopamine antagonist → used for treating schizophrenia (**negative symptoms**) → examples: **risperidone, olanzapine,** and **clozapine.** The atypical drugs have **fewer extrapyramidal symptoms** (EPS). They also cause sedation, QT prolongation, and weight gain.

Clozapine causes **agranulocytosis**.

Examples of extrapyramidal symptoms (EPS) are listed below:

1. Acute dystonia: patient has muscle spasms/contraction/stiffness (torticollis), tongue twisting, oculogyric crisis (shifting of the head and eyes); usually occurs few hours-days after treatment → treatment: **antihistamines (diphenhydramine)** or **anticholinergic (benztropine)**.

2. Akathisia: look for a patient with subjective feeling of restlessness, unable to sit still, and pacing around not being at ease; usually occurs few days after treatment → treatment: **beta blockers (propranolol)**, benzodiazepines, or anticholinergics.

3. Tardive dyskinesia: patients have facial/perioral movements including protruding of tongue, chewing, and grimacing; usually occurs **years** after treatment → treatment: **discontinue antipsychotic medication and use alternate medication such as an atypical antipsychotics** (clozapine)**.

4. Parkinsonism: also known as **dyskinesia** → patients have symptoms of Parkinson's disease such as **cogwheel rigidity**, mask-like face, drooling, shuffling gait, and stiffness; usually occurs **months** after treatment → treatment: **antihistamines (diphenhydramine)**, **anticholinergic (benztropine)**, or dopamine agonist (**amantadine**).

5. Neuroleptic malignant syndrome (NMS): a complication of antipsychotic medication which is also life-threatening. Patients present with muscular rigidity, obtundation, mutism, **high fever**, akinesia, dystonia, tachycardia, diaphoresis, and hypertension → labs will show **increased level of creatine phosphokinase (CPK)**, myoglobinuria, and increased LFTs → can worsen to rhabdomyolysis → treatment: discontinue antipsychotics, hydration, and **dantrolene**/bromocriptine.

Eating Disorders
Anorexia Nervosa

1. Most common in female teenagers with age-of-onset being 15, but can affect young adults too.
2. Findings: Overly concerned about weight (with body weight 15% below average), excessive dieting and exercising (**athlete**), amenorrhea, binge eating, and purging/vomiting.
3. Diagnosis: History and physical examination. Observe height and weight, and extremities for dry skin, fine hair, pallor, peripheral edema, and bradycardia. Obtain electrolytes, CBC, TFTs, LFTs, and ECG. Patients who are severely underweight/showing signs of dehydration should be hospitalized.

4. Treatment: Slowly increase calories consumption, SSRIs, and psychotherapy (individual, family, and group).

Bulimia Nervosa

1. Most common in female teenagers with age-of-onset being 15, but can affect young adults too.
2. Findings: Binge eating with lack of control results in purging (self-induced vomiting, excessive exercising, and laxative use), normal/overweight, **eroded tooth enamel,** and **eroded skin over the knuckles**.
3. Diagnosis: History and physical examination. Check electrolyes abnormalities (hypokalemia, hypochloremic, and metabolic alkalosis), CBC, and TFTs.
4. Treatment: Cognitive behavioral therapy (CBT) and antidepressants.

Suicide

1. Causes: Depression, loss of employment, single/divorce/widowed, or loss of a loved one/spouse.
2. Risk factors: **Prior suicide attempt** (best indicator of repeat suicide), substance abuse, male sex > 45 years of age, prior psychiatric disorder, and positive family history.
3. Men **commit** suicide four times more often than women; while women **attempt** suicide four times more often than men.

Personality Disorders

1. Paranoid: Patients who is distrustful and suspicious, and thinks everyone is after them. For example, they are distrustful of doctors who are actually trying to help them.

2. Schizoid: Patients are loners, isolated from everyone with no friends or social interaction.

3. Schizotypal: Patients have distorted perceptuals, bizarre beliefs, and magical thinking with no psychosis.

4. Histrionic: Patients are excessively dramatic/emotionally, attention-seeking, and manipulative. They also inppropriately sexually seductive towards others (usually

towards males).

5. Narcissistic: Patients show lack of empathy, sense of grandiosity and entitlement.

6. Borderline: Known as the 'split' personality where patients tend to change how they feel about people or certain things (they like; then they don't like). They also have unstable mood, relationships, and behavior; suicidal attempts, and impulsiveness.

7. Antisocial: Look for history of someone who is aggressive, conduct disorder as a child, violated the rights of others by torturing animals or have destroyed properties, and lack remorse. Associated with alcoholism and somatization disorder. Occurs around 18 years of age.

8. Avoidant: Patients have **fear of rejection** and of being disliked by others; so they **avoid** having people around or building friendships; although they would like to have friendships.

9. Obsessive-compulsive: not to be confused with OCD; patients are stubborn, controlling, and worry about being perfect with everything.

10. Dependent: Patients are very **submissive** and **dependent** on others (for example: their spouse) and cannot make decisions on their own. Usually seen in a wife who is dependent on her abusive husband.

Ethics
General

1. Do not tell a patient's employer or insurance about the patient's medical condition or diagnosis without getting a written permission from your patient.
2. Always respect a patient's wish on the do-not-resuscitates (DNRs).
3. A **competent** patient has the right to refuse treatment (even if it could lead to death). When a patient is **incompetent**, a surrogate decision-maker or health care power of attorney should be appointed by the court. If there is no surrogate decision-maker appointed yet, you may go with the family's wish if they all agree on the same wish. If there is a disagreement, obtain an ethics committee consult.
4. **Autonomy**: a patient's right to make a decision based on one's beliefs and morals.
5. **Informed consent**: discussing with a patient the diagnosis and prognosis of his/her medical condition while indicating the proposed treatment plan, its risk, and benefits of the treatment and/or other medical treatment option. **No diagnosis**

can be hidden from a patient. Respect a patient's decision when they ask that only certain information be shared with them.

6. The **treatment of a minor** < 18 years of age usually requires a parental consent **except** in the following situations: when a patient is emancipated (such as living alone, married, raising children, financially independent, or serving in the armed forces), requesting birth control, in treatment of sexually transmitted diseases (STDs), pregnancy, or psychiatry disorder.

7. The times that you **may break a patient's confidentiality** are as follows: when a court gives the order to do so, in suspected child abuse, in duty-to-warn and protect, in danger-to-others, and in reportable disease (such as gonorrhea, chlamydia, syphilis, tuberculosis, measles, rubella, or smallpox).

8. Restraints: you may use restraints on violent and psychiatric patients when they are a danger to themselves and others around them. **Endangerment to others** is another reason why you can **hospitalize a psychiatric patient against his/her own will**.

9. Do-not-resuscitates (DNRs): respect the wish of a patient in a DNR despite others' (family, caretaker) wishes.

10. Advance directives: statements from patients indicating what they want in resuscitative circumstances.

11. Pain management in terminally-ill patients: no patient deserves to suffer in pain; so give adequate pain medications when needed to alleviate pain. You may start with NSAIDs, but do not be reluctant to give narcotics when appropriate.

12. Withdrawal of treatment or care: may follow from a DNR wish of a patient, advance directive, family's wish, or a physician finding the need to do so (for example a physician may withdraw or withhold treatment in a suffering patient). A patient's DNR supercedes family's request. Whenever there is a disagreement between family members, seek ethics committee or court's decision.

13. Euthanasia: also known as physician-assisted suicide where the physician assists a competent patient to end his/her life through administration of drugs. It is illegal in United States except the state of Oregon.

PSYCHIATRY & ETHICS 1-LINER JUNKY CASES

- Depression can be due to a general medical condition such as substance abuse, stroke, or malignancy → and anxiety can be due to a condition such as hyperthyroidism, caffeine, or hypercalcemia.
- Cyclothymia => two or more years of **mild depression + hypomania**.
- Dysthymia => two or more years of **depressed 'mood' only** (no mania or psychosis).
- Do not hesitate to treat patients with major depression who are also presenting with **psychosis** → add antipsychotic to the antidepressant.
- Pseudodementia => in elderly patients, depression can mimic dementia → an event in the patient's life triggers depression which presents as dementia.
- Malingering => patient assumes a sick role and intentionally creates symptoms **seeking an external gain** (money or food).
- Factitious disorder => patient (**usually a healthcare worker**) assumes a sick role and intentionally creates symptoms **seeking a secondary gain** (leave from work).
- Homosexuality in any form is considered normal without any disease/pathology.
- Dissociative or psychogenic fugue => look for a patient who has amnesia, traveled, and assumed a new identity.
- Dissociative identity or multiple personality disorder => look for a patient with history of childhood sexual abuse who now has an identity problem.
- Delirium => frequently seen in hospitalized elderly patients with **acute flunctuations** (waxing and weaning effect during the day) in consciousness mimicking a psychological problem → look for change in medications, electrolyte imbalances, or infections.
- Dementia => chronic, irreversible process with normal consciousness → think of alzheimer's disease, vascular dementia, or Huntington's disease.
- **Narcolepsy** => a mood disorder that involves daytime sleepiness → presents as **decreased rapid eye movement (REM) latency, hypnagogic** (right before the patient falls asleep) **or hypnopompic** (right before the patient wakes up) **hallucinations, cataplexy** (sudden loss of muscle tone/sudden onset of sleep) → treatment: Amphetamine (**methylphenidate**) or non-amphetamine stimulant (**modafinil**).
- **Normal grief** => may appear similar to depression; however, there are **no suicidal ideation or feelings of worthlessness** in normal grief.
- **Serotonin syndrome** => results usually from taking MAOIs + SSRIs or SSRIs + atypical antipsychotics → presents with tachycardia, diaphoresis, delirium, hyperreflexia, and myoclonus → watch for hyperthermia, rhabdomyolysis, and seizures if severe → treatment: discontinue medications, supportive care and hydration; **cyproheptadine** may also help.

Chapter 17
Immunology
Hypersensitivity Reactions

1. Type I hypersensitivity: This type of hypersensitivity involves the anaphylactic reaction where the release of histamine from cells such as mast cells and basophils is as a result of IgE antibodies → some of the examples include: allergies such as with foods and medications (penicillin and sulfa drugs), anaphylaxis associated with bee stings, atopy, asthma, allergic rhinitis, urticaria, and hay fever → **Findings:** look for a patient during the winter season who has rhinorrhea, and the nostrils are pale, blue, and sometimes the nasal turbinates may be edematous. Patients with bee stings may appear more ill, and present with dyspnea, wheezing, urticaria, and edema of the larynx → **diagnosis: increased IgE, eosinophils, C1 esterase inhibitor deficiency** (a complement, to diagnose family history of **hereditary angioedema** => autosomal dominant and **decreased C2** and **C4 complement levels**) → **treatment:** in anaphylaxis = **subcutaneous epinephrine (1:1000)** +/- steroids and diphenhydramine (antihistamine); and in hereditary angioedema = C1 esterase inhibitor, **fresh frozen plasma (FFP)**, **ecallantide** (maintenance in chronic cases) and **danazol** (androgen).

2. Type II hypersensitivity: This type of hypersensitivity involves the cytotoxic reaction where the pre-formed IgG and IgM make a reaction that results in an inflammatory process → some of the examples include: autoimmune hemolytic anemia, transfusion reactions, hyperacute transplant rejection, Goodpasture syndrome, ITP, and autoimmune diseases like Graves disease or pernicious anemia → **Findings:** look for a patient who is having a reaction to a kidney transplant or hemolysis → **diagnosis:** based on the disease causing the hypersensitivity, but may include **Coomb's test** (for autoimmune hemolytic anemia) → **treatment:** depends on the cause.

3. Type III hypersensitivity: This type of hypersensitivity involves the immune complex-mediated reaction where the antigen-antibody complexes are deposited in blood vessels thereby causing inflammatory processes → some of the examples include serum sickness, glomerulonephritis, cryoglobulinemia, autoimmune diseases, and lupus.

4. Type IV hypersensitivity: This type of hypersensitivity involves the delayed reaction where sensitized T lymphocytes release inflammatory processes → some of the examples include contact dermatitis (nickel and poison ivy), tuberculin skin test, sarcoidosis, and chronic kidney transplant rejection.

Kidney Transplant Rejection:

1. Hyperacute transplant rejection: occurs anytime from **minutes to hours** → due to **preformed antibodies**, and it is B-cell mediated (patient's serum has preformed anti-donor antibodies).

2. Acute transplant rejection: occurs anytime from days to weeks → T-cell mediated immune response.

3. Chronic transplant rejection: occurs anytime from months to years.

IMMUNOLOGY 1-LINER JUNKY CASES

- Tacrolimus inhibits the activation of T helper cells.
- **Allergic rhinitis**: look for rhinorrhea, congestion, sneezing, nasal itching + history of asthma → treatment: avoid allergens, nasal saline spray, antihistamine (fexofenadine), **intranasal corticosteroid** (most effective), pseudoephedrine, cromolyn, intranasal anticholinergic (ipratropium bromide), and immunotherapy +/- desensitization.
- Common variable immunodeficiency (CVID) => occurs between 20-30 years of age with **recurrent sinopulmonary infections** and **malabsorption disorder** → diagnosis: low levels of Igs → treatment: IV immunoglobulins (IVIGs) → there is risk of lymphoma and autoimmune disease.
- IgA deficiency => **most common immunodeficiency** in U.S. → look for a patient who develops anaphylaxis reaction after obtaining blood transfusion → patients may also have **malabsorption disorder** and **URIs/recurrent sinopulmonary infections** → treatment: antibiotics (for URI).
- Bruton's X-linked agammaglobulinemia => is X-linked recessive disorder that usually presents in boys after 6 months of age, but may present earlier → diagnosis: **low or absent of B cells**, quantitative Ig levels + **recurrent URIs/sinopulmonary infections** → treatment: IV immunoglobulins (IVIGs).
- IgE syndrome => look for *S. aureus* causes skin infections.

Chapter 18
Rheumatology
Rheumatoid Arthritis

---

1. Rheumatoid arthritis is the chronic, symmetrical inflammation of the joints affecting women between 20-50 years of age.
2. Findings: patients usually present with low-grade fever, malaise, weight loss, **morning stiffness**, tender and swollen joints with subcutaneous nodules, and pannus (means presence of granulation tissue). Some patients may have other systemic symptoms such as pericarditis or pleural effusion, carpal tunnel syndrome, atlantoaxial joint subluxation, baker's cyst rupture, **swan neck, ulna deviation**, and boutonniere deformities.
3. Diagnosis: start with rheumatoid factor (positive in 75% of patients) with the following criteria: **prolonged morning stiffness for more than 1 hour** (worse in the morning and improves as the day progresses), arthritis affect at least three joints including the hands (examples are **MCP, PIP**, ankle, and **wrist**), rheumatoid nodules, x-rays of affected joints (look for erosions), **joint aspiration (WBCs > 2000)**, and **anti-citrullinated cyclic peptide (CCP)** (has 95% specificity).
4. Treatment: begin with NSAIDs +/- hydroxychloroquine; **prednisone** (for flare-ups; second-line); if severe, add **methotrexate,** then etanercept/infliximab (anti-TNF treatment). Immunosuppressants are used when everything else fails.

Osteoarthritis

---

1. Osteoarthritis is a chronic disease with minimal or no inflammation of the joints. Usually affects older patients; therefore, incidence increases with age. Also associated with obesity.
2. Etiology: due to prolonged history of arthritis, advanced age, obesity, and trauma.
3. Findings: Joint pain without inflammation, pain worsens during the day or in the evening with activity and improves with rest; may involve the hip, knees, and spine; **bony** spurs, and the **Bouchard nodes** are found at the proximal interphalangeal (**PIP**) joint and the **Heberden nodes** are at the distal interphalangeal (**DIP**) joint.
4. Diagnosis: History and physical, x-ray (shows joint-space narrowing with osteophytes), normal (calcium and phosphate), and WBCs < 2000.
5. Treatment: Weight loss, low-impact exercise/quadriceps strengthening exercise, NSAIDs or **acetaminophen** (use initially for mild pain); then **intra-articular**

---

corticosteroids (for mild-moderate pain), and joint replacement (for severe and disabling symptoms). Other treatment may include chondroitin, tramadol, and lidocaine patches.

Systemic Lupus Erythematous (SLE)

1. SLE is an autoimmune disease leading to chronic inflammatory and multisystem disorders. It is commonly seen in women from ages 20-50.
2. Findings: important features include malar rash (butterfly rash on the mid-face), **discoid rash** (scaly papules), **photosensitive rash**, arthritis, **oral ulcers**, fatigue, weight loss, fever, anemia, thrombocytopenia, and kidney failure. Some patients may have other systemic symptoms such as pericarditis, pulmonary hypertension, pleural effusion, and pericardial effusion. Neurological symptoms may include headaches, seizures, depression, and psychosis.
3. Diagnosis: start with antinuclear antibody (**ANA**; highly sensitive), **anti-dsDNA** (highly specific), **anti-Smith antibody** (highly specific), positive syphilis test (Venereal Disease Research Laboratory or rapid plasma reagin); anticardiolipin and positive lupus anticoagulant (to check for antiphospholipid antibody syndrome), **decreased complements C3 and C4**, and **increased CRP/ESR**.
4. Treatment: NSAIDs (initially; for arthritis), hydroxychloroquine (used when NSAIDs fail; for arthritis and rashes), **steroids** (for flare-ups), and immunosuppressants. Steroids, **mycophenolate mofetil** (preferred for renal-nephritis), or cyclophosphamide helps the renal function. It is important to treat **antiphospholipid syndrome** patients with **lifelong wafarin therapy** to prevent thrombotic events.
5. **Complications**: Spontaneous abortion, congenital block, and thrombosis due to antiphospholipid syndrome.

Gout

1. Gout is the intra-articular deposition of monosodium urate crystals into the joints which usually presents at nights as 'acute attacks'. Attacks are precipitated by alcohol, diuretics (thiazides), **chlorthalidone**, and **nicotinic acid**.
2. Findings: look for a patient, usually **obese/alcoholic**, who complains of **severe pain** (sensitive to the touch), **erythematous/redness**, and **swelling** that wakes patient up from sleep, **podagra** (patient's great toes have uric acid deposited), and **tophi** (shows subcutaneous uric acid deposits). Tophi may lead to joint deformation.
3. Diagnosis: some acute attacks are triggered by diets; so watch for patients who

consume high purine diets (such as alcohol and red meat), diuretics, chlorthalidone, nicotinic acid, and cyclosporine. Joint aspiration (**athrocentesis shows needle-shaped crystals with negative birefringence**), increased serum uric acid, 24-hour urine collection of uric acid, and x-rays (shows punched-out lesions/erosions).

4. Treatment: avoid high purine diets, weight loss, NSAIDs (indomethacin) or colchicine (for acute attacks), steroids (second-line for acute attacks), and allopurinol/probenecid or sulfinpyrazone (**not for acute attacks, but for prevention/maintenance**). Also **febuxostat** (xanithineoxidase inhibitor) has been used when allopurinol fails.

5. **Complications**: Chronic urate nephropathy and nephrolithiasis.

Pseudogout

1. Findings: Similar to gout, but affects predominantly the **knees**.
2. Diagnosis: Joint aspiration (**athrocentesis shows rhomboid-shaped calcium pyrophosphate dihydrate crystals with positive birefringence**).
3. Treatment: NSAIDs (indomethacin) or colchicine (not as effective in pseudogout compared to gout), and steroids (second-line for acute attacks).

Ankylosing Spondylitis

1. Family history with chronic back pain and **worsening morning stiffness and gradually improves after activity** → usually occurs in men between the ages of 20-45.
2. Findings: Chronic back pain, sacroilitis, and arthritis. Other symptoms may include **uveitis**, fever, anemia, aortitis, dactylitis, plantar fasciitis, **restriction of chest wall expansion** and spinal mobility.
3. Diagnosis: **Associated with HLA-B27**. X-ray of the lumbar spine (shows "bamboo spine"), AP pelvic x-ray (shows sclerosis of the sacroiliac joints and pseudowidening with erosions). MRI is **most sensitive**.
4. Treatment: Exercise and NSAIDs.

- **Reiter syndrome**: is also associated with **HLA-B27** → syndrome presents with urethritis from (chlamydial infection), conjunctivitis, and arthritis. Other symptoms are uveitis and penile ulcers. Treatment of arthritis is NSAIDs and urethritis is azithromycin for patient and partner. Patient may have GI infection instead of urethritis (Chlamydia infection).

Scleroderma

1. Progressive and symmetrical thickening of the skin common in young adults to older women.
2. Findings: **CREST** symptoms include **c**alcinosis, **R**aynaud phenomenon, **e**sophageal dysmotility, **s**clerodactyly, **t**elangiectasias. Look for complaints of tightening of the face and heartburn. **Other type of skin involvement is 'diffuse'** which is rapid and a generalized form with risk of progression to **pulmonary hypertension** and **kidney failure** which can be confirmed with **anti-Scl-70 antibody** (for diffuse form).
3. Diagnosis: ANA (for screening), **anticentromere antibody** (confirmatory test for CREST), and **antitopoisomerase** (confirmatory test for scleroderma).
4. Treatment: Steroids. Use **sildenafil or bosentan** to treat pulmonary hypertension. Don't use sildenafil until 24 hours after taking nitroglycerin.

Sjogren Syndrome

1. An autoimmune disease causing dry/gritty eyes (keratoconjunctivitis sicca), dry mouth (xerostomia).
2. Diagnosis: Positive lip biopsy, slit-lamp exam, schirmer's test, salivary gland ultrasound, salivary scintigraphy, chest x-ray, **anti-SS-A (Ro)**, and **anti-SS-B (La)**.
3. Treatment: Eye drops (to keep eyes moistened), pilocarpine, **cevimiline** (increases eye and oral secretions), NSAIDs, hydroxychloroquine, cyclophosphamide, and surgery.
4. Complication: Risk of lymphoma.

Polymyositis

1. Inflammation of the proximal muscles which occurs mainly in older women of ages 50-70.
2. Findings: Symmetrical proximal muscle weakness and pain with patient complaint of difficulty rising from a chair +/- dyspnea.
3. Diagnosis: **increased [ESR, CPK, and aldolase], EMG** (shows fibrillations), and **muscle biopsy** (shows muscle degeneration and inflammation). The presence of **anti-Jo 1 antibodies** also indicates **interstitial lung disease**.
4. Treatment: Steroids.

- **Dermatomyositis:** 33% of patients with polymyositis have dermatomyositis which is the skin involvement → with symptoms of heliotrope rash (violaceous perioribital rash), shawl sign (erythema on the shoulder and neck region), and Gottron's papules of the hands → **risk of malignancy!**

Polymyalgia Rheumatica

1. Inflammation of the muscles involving the pectoral, pelvic girdles, and sometimes the neck which occurs mostly in older women around 50 years of age.
2. Findings: Tender and stiffness of the pectoral/shoulder and pelvic girdles, fatigue, fever, weight loss, anemia, and malaise. **Patients complain of inability to raise hands/arms above their heads or cannot comb their hair.**
3. Diagnosis: **Increased ESR** and anemia.
4. Treatment: **Prednisone** (low-dose)**.**

Temporal Arteritis

1. Also known as the giant cell arteritis, and it is related to polymyalgia rheumatica → involves the **central retinal artery**.
2. Findings: jaw pain, temporal headache and tenderness, weight loss, myalgia, and fever.
3. Diagnosis: **Increased ESR usually around 100**, eye exam (**urgently,** refer to ophthalmologist to prevent risk of **blindness**), and temporal artery biopsy (confirms).
4. Treatment: **Prednisone (high-dose).**
5. **Complication: Blindness!**

Fibromyalgia

1. Non-inflammatory changes of different muscle groups commonly in young adult to older women.
2. Findings: Fatigue, myalgias, muscle weakness, **depression**, and **tender muscles on palpation affecting at least 11 of 18 trigger points**. Watch also for patients with stress and irritable bowel syndrome (IBS).
3. Diagnosis: Normal labs (ESR, muscle biopsy, and EMG).
4. Treatment: NSAIDs, exercise, **pregablin,** transcutaneous electrical nerve stimulation, psychotherapy, SSRIs, and relaxation/stress reduction techniques.

Paget Disease

1. Bone pathology showing breakdown of bone and regeneration affecting mostly older men.
2. Findings: **complaint of wearing larger-sized hats**, bone disease affecting the pelvic and skull and causing **pain** and **arthritis**.
3. Diagnosis: **Increased alkaline phosphatase**, but **normal levels of calcium and phosphorus.** Urinalysis shows increased hydroxyproline and roentengram studies show dense and enlarged bones. Bone scan may also be obtained.
4. Treatment: NSAIDs initially (for pain), bisphosphonate (for severe disease), and calcitonin.
5. **Complications**: **nerve deafness** and **osteosarcoma**.

Lower Back Pain

1. Ankylosing spondylitis: Lower back pain that is worsen in the morning with stiffness and improves with use → affects the sacroiliac joints, knees, and the hips → diagnosis: lumbar spine x-ray, AP pelvic x-ray, and MRI.
2. Cauda equina: A medical emergency that causes bladder and bowel incontinence, and saddle anesthesia → diagnosis: **STAT MRI!**
3. Spinal stenosis: Chronic pain in the lower back that worsens with standing/walking and improves with sitting or leaning forward → diagnosis: MRI.
4. Myofascial strain: Secondary to trauma → presents with **perispinal tenderness** → diagnosis: MRI → treatment: NSAIDs.

RHEUMATOLOGY 1-LINER JUNKY CASES

- Anti-TNF (etanercept) => risk of infections → check PPD test + hepatitis B and C before the treatment of rheumatoid arthritis.
- Felty syndrome => rheumatoid arthritis + splenomegaly + neutropenia.
- Methotrexate is not recommended for use in pregnancy, HIV, liver disease, kidney damage, or bone marrow suppression patients.
- Juvenile arthritis => myalgia + fever + **salmon rash** + lymphadenopathy → diagnosis: **negative** (ANA, RF), increased WBCs, and **increased ferritin**.
- Avoid allopurinol during acute gout attacks due to worsening of symptoms.
- Watch for charcot joints in diabetics presenting with peripheral neuropathy and deformities due to excessive use of the joints.
- Plantar fasciitis => pain on plantar side of the foot that **resolves** with walking → treatment: spontaneous recovery + stretching.
- Tarsal tunnel syndrome => pain on plantar side of the foot that **worsens** with walking + numbness → treatment: steroid injection at site, then surgery.
- **Takayasu arteritis** => occurs in Asian young women → they present with difficulty to assess pulse and blood pressure, aorta and carotid (may cause stroke) arteries are affected → diagnosis: angiogram → treatment: steroids +/- cyclophosphamide.
- Polyarteritis nodosa => vasculitis affecting medium-sized vessels → Findings: abdominal pain, fever, anemia, weight loss, hematuria, pericarditis, and peripheral neuropathies → associated with hepatitis B → diagnosis: biopsy (shows vasculitis of vessels; for example, the vessels of the abdomen).
- Behcet syndrome => usually presents with a male young adult man with tender oral and genital lesions/ulcers, optic neuritis/uveitis, arthritis, and look for a patient with increased sensitivity to sites of needle injections → treatment: steroids, colchicines, and cyclophosphamide → complication: blindness (due to eye involvement) + abscess (at injection sites).
- Gonococcal arthritis => painful, swollen knee, fever, and **leukocytosis with a left shift**.
- **Septic arthritis** => anthrocentesis has **> 75,000 WBCs** + fever + severe pain + **reduced range of motion** + large effusion → treatment: IV ceftriaxone + vancomycin.
- For gout, gonococcal arthritis, or septic arthritis, treat with anthrocentesis (joint aspiration).
- Metastatic bone pain can be treated with NSAIDs initially if the pain is mild to moderate, then you may use narcotics.
- Eosinophilic fasciitis => presents like scleroderma → look for **increased eosinophils + peau d'orange (orange peel)** → treatment: steroids.
- **Cryoglobulinemia** => associated with hepatitis **C** + kidney problems → look for skin involvement + arthritis + malaise → treatment: interferon + ribavirin (for

hepatitis C).

- **Baker's cyst** => associated with rheumatoid arthritis → diagnosis: ultrasound (to rule out DVT) → NSAIDs and steroids injection at site.
- **Muscular dystrophy** => due to defects in coding for structural proteins → patients usually have difficulty in climbing the stairs → diagnosis: creatine kinase.

Chapter 19
Ophthalmology
Retinal Detachment

1. Findings: presents as 'floaters' or 'curtain veil' over patient's eyes.
2. Diagnosis: a medical emergency that requires consult with ophthalmologist for eye/retinal exam.
3. Treatment: a medical emergency; **head tilt** while you obtain ophthalmologist consult to prevent loss of vision includes **surgery (reattachment of the retina)**.

Closed-angle Glaucoma

1. Sudden visual decreased/loss due to increased intraocular pressure (> 25 mmHg).
2. Findings: painful eye, fixed & dilated pupil, nausea/vomiting, pink-red eye, and halos around lights.
3. Diagnosis: increased intraocular pressure.
4. Treatment: emergent ophthalmologist referral to prevent loss of vision; pilocarpine, timolol, or acetazolamide.

Open-angle Glaucoma

1. Gradual loss of vision due to increased intraocular pressure (< 25 mmHg).
2. Findings: **painless eye** and elevated cup-to-disk ratio.
3. Diagnosis: increased intraocular pressure and funduscopic exam shows elevated cup-to-disk ratio.
4. Treatment: non-emergency; treat with pilocarpine, timolol, or acetazolamide.

Central Retinal Vein Occlusion

1. Sudden visual loss that is usually due to other underlying disorders such as diabetes, hypertension, and malignancy.
2. Findings: painless, unilateral, sudden visual loss.
3. Diagnosis: funduscopic exam.

4. Treatment: supportive.

Central Retinal Artery Occlusion

1. Sudden visual loss that is usually due to an emboli. Associated with **temporal arteritis**.
2. Findings: painless, unilateral, sudden visual loss, pale fundus, and **red spot** in the macular.
3. Diagnosis: funduscopic exam.
4. Treatment: supportive (such as **ocular massage**).

Macular Degeneration

1. Causes blindness.
2. Findings: painless, bilateral, gradual visual loss.
3. Diagnosis: funduscopic exam shows drusen deposits.
4. Treatment: there is no beneficial management available.

Cataracts

1. Gradual visual loss (most common). Associated with the use of steroids.
2. Findings: painless, bilateral/unilateral, gradual visual loss, and **absent red reflex**.
3. Diagnosis: funduscopic exam.
4. Treatment: surgery.

OPHTHALMOLOGY 1-LINER JUNKY CASES

- Central retinal artery occlusion → associated with an emboli → presents with pale fundus + 'cherry-red spot' seen in the macular.
- Uveitis => diagnosis: **slit-lamp exam** → treatment: corticosteroids.
- Conjunctivitis => categorized into chemical (look for history of chemical spill/use), viral (**itchy, watery eye, preauricular lymphadenopathy**), bacterial (**purulent**), and allergic (**similar to viral**, but **no lymphadenopathy**) → treatment: irrigation (chemical), conservative (viral), topical sulfacetamide +/- topical erythromycin and IV ceftriaxone (bacterial; for *Nisseria gonorrhea*)*; and doxycyline for *Chlamydia trachomatis*).

Index

www.ingramcontent.com/pod-product-compliance
Lightning Source LLC
Chambersburg PA
CBHW081524220326
41598CB00036B/6317